PRAISE FOR MACKIE SHILSTONE

"Mackie's system helped me boost my stamina, strength, and speed, and it prolonged my career. I don't know where I'd be without it."

—OZZIE SMITH, FORMER ALL-STAR, ST. LOUIS CARDINALS

"Mackie's been the difference. He helped me get my weight down and strengthen my whole body. I've been All-Pro every year I've trained with him."

—LOMAS BROWN, NEW YORK GIANTS

"Mackie is one of my secret weapons."

—WILL CLARK, ST. LOUIS CARDINALS

"I could go anywhere, but I choose to train with Mackie Shilstone."

—BRETT BUTLER, FORMER LOS ANGELES DODGERS PLAYER

"It's like we found a gold mine. We've seen injuries go down and performance go up."

—AL ROSEN, FORMER GENERAL MANAGER, SAN FRANCISCO GIANTS

"Mackie has been at the forefront of fitness and conditioning with his unique ability to integrate sport-specific training methods that fit the individual athlete's needs."

—MARK A. LETENDRE, A.T.C., DIRECTOR OF UMPIRE MEDICAL SERVICES
FOR MAJOR LEAGUE BASEBALL

"He adds years to your career."

—MORTEN ANDERSEN, ATLANTA FALCONS

"When the Royals send players to Mackie Shilstone, we are always confident that they will return in better athletic condition, with a better understanding of how to stay in shape throughout the course of their careers."

—JAY HINRICHS, VICE PRESIDENT OF ADMINISTRATION AND DEVELOPMENT,
KANSAS CITY ROYALS

"Mackie Shilstone has worked wonders with my clients. He's on the cutting edge of strength and conditioning for professional athletes, and I encourage all my clients to work with him whenever possible."
—MARK BARTELSTEIN, MARK BARTELSTEIN AND ASSOCIATES

"Mackie Shilstone's program really saved my life (literally). . . . I lost a total of 34 pounds over a 2½ month period. A by-product of the testing found that I had high blood sugar, high cholesterol, and some potential heart problems could have been in my future. Through Mackie's persistence, he provided me with clinical help that will allow me to have a long and prosperous life."
—JOHN "ROCKY" ROE, UMPIRE, MAJOR LEAGUE BASEBALL

"At night, I used to feel worn out because my energy level would just be gone. But I feel revitalized and have a lot of energy since I've been on this program."
—DON, TEACHER AND COACH

"I was never hungry. There were two snacks and three meals a day. I probably ate more on this than on any other diet, and I probably ate right."
—JERRY, POLICE OFFICER

"Mackie's approach to fitness and performance enhancement is first-rate."
—JOHN G. QUIGLEY, MANAGING PARTNER, NASSAU CAPITAL, PRINCETON, NEW JERSEY

Lose Your Love Handles

A 3-STEP PROGRAM TO STREAMLINE YOUR WAIST IN 30 DAYS

Mackie Shilstone

A Perigee Book

A Perigee Book
Published by The Berkley Publishing Group
A division of Penguin Putnam Inc.
375 Hudson Street
New York, New York 10014

Copyright © 2001 by Mackie Shilstone, Inc.
Text design by Pauline Neuwirth
Cover design by Dawn Velez Le'Bron
Cover photo copyright © Super Stock, Inc.
Interior photos copyright © Judy Johnson
Interior illustrations by Barbara Siede

First edition: April 2001

Published simultaneously in Canada.

The Penguin Putnam Inc. World Wide Web site address is
http: //www.penguinputnam.com

Library of Congress Cataloging-in-Publication Data
Shilstone, Mackie.
    Lose your love handles : a 3-step program to streamline your waist in 30 days / Mackie Shilstone.
        p.cm.
    Includes index.
    ISBN 0-399-52660-9
        1. Weight loss. 2. Glycemic index. 3. Insulin resistance. 4. Exercise for men. 5. Reducing
    exercises. I. Title.

RM222.2 .S5268 2000
613.7'0449—dc21   00-061185

Printed in the United States of America
10 9 8 7

DISCLAIMER: Every effort has been made to ensure that the information contained in this book is complete and accurate. However, neither the publisher nor the author is engaged in rendering professional advice or services to the individual reader. The ideas, procedures, and suggestions contained in this book are not intended as a substitute for consulting with your physician. All matters regarding your health require medical supervision. Neither the author nor the publisher shall be liable or responsible for any loss, injury, or damage allegedly arising from any information or suggestion in this book.

CONTENTS

ACKNOWLEDGMENTS

I wish to offer my deep gratitude and sincere appreciation to the following people:

My loving wife and best friend, Sandy, who has the patience of Job and provided her support to help all of my efforts to be realized.

To my collaborator, Joy Parker, for the time and effort she gave to this project. Joy's ability to comprehend and interpret complicated medical technology and terminology was such that she was able to present this in an easy-to-understand format. Joy has been able to get into my head and translate my thoughts into the written word. I would not even think about having anyone else write for me in any future publication or book other than Joy Parker.

To my agent, Bonnie Solow, who worked very hard and long hours to do her best for me and who never quits. Bonnie is truly the best representative any person could ever want. She commands tremendous respect in her field, which is earned through dedication, commitment, and a thorough knowledge of her industry.

To Judy Johnson for her endless patience and good humor as this book and its programs went through many, many refinements.

Acknowledgments

To Dr. Ann de Wees Allen, Doctor of Naturopathy and a prominent scientist and researcher with the Glycemic Research Institute in Washington, D.C. Dr. Allen graciously allowed me to interview her for the book and provided me with much essential information, including permission to use the list of glycemically acceptable and unacceptable foods that she has developed.

To Brian Picou and Kat Bradley for compiling the statistics on the six men who participated in the study and patiently keeping track of their progress for 3 months. Thanks especially to Brian, who always patiently provided me with up-to-the minute data.

To Molly Kimball for the excellent work she did in providing delicious food plans and for her helpful comments on the draft of chapter 3.

To Jim Flarity, Ph.D., for being available to clarify important medical questions in the text.

To George Stylianides, Ph.D., for your help in capturing the dynamics of racewalking in the illustration in chapter 4.

To Barbara Seide, my illustrator, who patiently worked with me to provide excellent and helpful drawings for the manuscript.

To Mike Derrington, Product Manager of Personal Edge, a Dupont Company, and a longtime friend and supporter, for his assistance with cutting edge nutritional technology.

For Ken Kachtik, general manager of The Elmwood Fitness Center in New Orleans, who had the insight to create the Mackie Shilstone Center for Performance Enhancement and Lifestyle Management and the commitment to stand behind it. He is a true friend.

I also wish to thank all of the men who participated in the test pilot of this program, especially Jerry Ursin, Donald Thomas, Robert Nelson, Stan Stopa, Robert Italiano, and Dorian Bennett.

To Dr. Gerry Provance, my chiropractor, who gave me appropriate insight into dynamic pelvic stabilization and the appropriate exercises to achieve it safely and effectively.

To Dr. Merv Trail, chancellor of Louisiana State University Health Sciences Center and Dr. Charles Brown, Medical Director at the Center for Sports Performance Fitness and Welleness, for their academic and moral support.

To our wonderful editor, Sheila Curry Oakes, for her insightful comments on the manuscript that helped us to take the book to another level of excellence. Thank you also, Sheila, for patiently answering all of our many questions.

FOREWORD
by Ozzie Smith

I played major league baseball for nineteen years. It had always been my goal to try and play effectively for as long as I could, but I believe my career would have been a lot shorter without the help and coaching of Mackie Shilstone.

Back in 1985, I felt that I only had a few more years to go in the game, and I decided I wanted to be known not just as a great defensive shortstop, but as a great all-around player. At the time, my batting average was only about .249, and I wasn't even considered a hitting threat. I needed to find a way to get bigger and stronger because, at 144 pounds, I didn't have a whole lot of size. I had heard about this guy Mackie Shilstone from Manute Bol, and I decided to see if he could help me.

When I began to train with Mackie, I felt that things really started to come together for me, both offensively and defensively. I had always worked hard with weights in the off-season, but I had never incorporated a good nutritional program to supplement weight lifting. Consequently, I would have a good first half of the season, but with my size I wasn't able to hold on to what I'd gained during a grueling 162-game schedule. By the time the second half rolled around, I was out of gas. I needed to figure out a way to keep the added weight and strength, and Mackie helped me to achieve my objective through his program of weight training and nutrition.

When I told Mackie I needed to get a lot bigger, he said to me, "I know you are a great defensive player. That's what your contract is based on. What if I waved a magic wand and gave you a lot more pounds, but you lost your agility and couldn't be a great defensive shortstop anymore? Would you really want what you got, even if you become a good hitter? I think our goal should be to design a program that will maintain your Gold Glove level and yet help you to be a better hitter."

And that's exactly what he did. Although Mackie had never worked with a baseball player before, he used his training and experience with many types of athletes to create a program for me with exercises that were very baseball specific. It was a learning experience for both of us. Trying to get that balance between the speed and agility I needed as a defensive shortstop, and the greater muscle and weight that I needed to become a better all-around player took some doing. I tipped the scales a few times. As I built muscle, my friends began calling me "Bulldog" because I'd gained so much weight, my neck was thicker, and I had muscles everywhere. They gave me a hard time, teasing me about that.

Mackie's knowledge base of what I was trying to accomplish, and his knowledge of human anatomy was amazing in itself. We would sit with doctors at lunchtime, and he would talk to them in their own language. In many instances doctors were asking *him* what he had experienced when he used certain products and supplements. That's basically the way we built up my muscles, by using amino acids and adding calories. Eating healthy calories along with doing weight lifting and sport-specific exercises allowed me to play a lot longer than I had anticipated.

I worked extremely hard with Mackie, and it paid off. That year I won the silver bat, with a batting average of .309. I went on to get eight gold gloves after that.

One of the impressive things about Mackie is that he isn't a person who says, "Hey, this is what I want *you* to do." He works out right along with you. I don't know exactly how many people he was training while he was working with me, but I know his plate was full. He was going all day. Sometimes when I'd go down to New Orleans and meet him in the morning, he would have already been up and worked out, or worked out somebody else before he and I even got started. His approach to what he does is all-out. He not only tells you how to do it, he *shows* you. He does it with you.

Mackie is an incredible motivator. He doesn't just train you to enhance your performance and be a better athlete, he gives you things that you can take with you for life—how to eat healthy, for example. When I first started to work his program, I saw changes so quickly that I felt inspired to continue. That's the trouble with most people, staying motivated. If you are trying to lose weight, for example, and you see yourself beginning to lose fat and build muscle within the first two or three days of being on the program, it gets you fired up. I picked up 7 to 10 pounds of muscle within the first few days of working with Mackie. That was amazing to me. Mackie explained it to me this way. The body, over the years, becomes depleted of certain things. For me, I lacked a proper amount of certain important amino acids, the building blocks of the body that help it to repair muscle tissue. We used those as the core of my supplementation program. I took them on a regular basis as I diligently worked out. When I saw results so quickly, I thought, "Oh, boy, we've got something here." It was a great experience and I stayed with Mackie for 11 years, from 1985 until I retired in 1996.

Mackie is one of the greatest human beings I have ever had a chance to meet. He's a very interesting person, and his knowledge base is unlimited. When he was training me, we were always joking around, in competition with each other. We used to throw the medicine ball a lot, and we'd tried to throw the ball right through each other. He'd talk about how hard his stomach was and how he was in much better shape than I was, and it would inspire me to work harder. I've enjoyed the time that I've had with Mackie. He's a great guy to work with, and it's been fun.

INTRODUCTION

I decided to write this book because, up to this point, no one has found a solution to reducing abdominal fat in men. Even though gaining weight in the "love handle" area is a classic, male fat pattern, the core area of the body has always been considered the most difficult to tone and reduce. When you walk down the streets of any town or city, you can see how many men over the age of 40—and even younger, as obesity is on the rise in America—have their stomachs protruding out over their belt buckles. Over the last twenty years as I have worked with over a thousand top athletes—boxers, men in the NFL, and professional baseball players—and thousands of ordinary men at my Center for Performance Enhancement and Lifestyle Management at the Elmwood Fitness Center in New Orleans, I have noticed a pattern. *Even when men train or work out on a regular basis, they* still *have difficulty reducing the love handle area.*

Because abdominal fat predisposes men to serious health risks, such as type 1 and type 2 diabetes, hypertension, and heart disease, I became determined to discover what physical processes and lifestyle choices were behind this fat gain. My timing was right on because I was able to find many recent scientific studies that had made breakthroughs in understanding these processes and how to counteract them. This research dovetailed beautifully with what I had observed in my work with athletes and the men at my gym. I had gotten results, and now I was beginning to understand why—and how to better teach men to get those results themselves.

In men, the largest proportion of extra fat gets stored in the abdominal area. When we do not exercise and when we eat too much of the wrong kinds of food, as that food is digested, we end up with more glucose in our blood than we can possibly use as fuel. When a person becomes overfat, he becomes insulin resistant. His cells get out of shape and lose much of their ability to respond to insulin. This leaves a surplus of glucose floating around in the body, much more than is necessary for its immediate metabolic needs. This, in turn, stimulates the pancreas to produce even more insulin to do its job of transporting this glucose into the cells. Since there are more fat cells in the abdomen of a man with a large waistline than anywhere else in his body, much of this fat ends up there. This creates a vicious circle, causing even more weight gain. The more fat you have, the more nutrients will be stored as fat.

Our caveman ancestors, who were much more physically active than we are and ate many more "complex" foods that digest slowly, such as lean meat, fibrous vegetables, and whole grains, burned much of their food as fuel in their daily living. Men today are more likely to be sitting behind a desk or standing next to a machine in a factory. Our high fat and high sugar, highly processed American diet only makes matters worse. Even our children are becoming more and more obese. This situation is only going to get worse because, as a society, we are becoming less and less active.

The good news is that when we eat the right kinds of low-glycemic foods, in the proper proportions of 55 percent low glycemic carbohydrates, 20 percent lean protein, and 25 percent acceptable fat, we can normalize our insulin response. By doing exercises that are specifically targeted to work the core area of the body, we can tone and firm that area and decrease the circumference of our waistline. Better yet, because the love handle area is one of the body's first choices for storing fat in men, it is also the first choice of fat to burn as fuel during exercise. This is what I call the "law of first in, first out."

I felt there was a need for a book about spot reducing in the love handle area because I wanted to take advantage of all of the newest research on health benefits, nutrition, and the advantages of aerobic and core exercises. I also felt that writing this book was a personal challenge. I've made my mark in all the areas that I have worked in as a performance management specialist. For nearly two decades, I've trained world-class athletes to perform better, with more focus, and maintain a healthier, balanced lifestyle. I have helped them to reach new levels of peak performance and achieve even greater success at what they already do best. Most important, I have helped them to stay on top by devising performance longevity programs that have extended by years the careers of professional athletes, even those in the body-destroying NFL, where the average career expectancy is only 3 to 5 years.

In *Lose Your Love Handles,* I hope to have an impact on the lifestyles of the man on the street. I want to be remembered as an individual who has changed the course of the way that we address our most serious risk factor for health and life extension, abdominal fat. I know this program is effective because of the tremendous results achieved by the six test subjects in chapter 6, who represent a diverse cross section of the population. I asked them to take on this program at the toughest time of the year—during Thanksgiving, Christmas, and Hanukkah. Their commitment to the program was based on their belief in and commitment to me. However, they stayed with the program during the stressful holidays because they began to see results. They saw changes in their bodies, felt better, and were told by friends and family members that they were looking better. I have also tested this program on members of the New Orleans Police Department, and the results have been outstanding.

One month is a realistic time period in which to see some kinds of results. I am asking my readers to pay particular attention to one particular statistic: the waist measurement. I use this variable because your scale weight will go up and down, but the waistline never lies. When you follow my three-fold plan of low-glycemic meals, aerobic exercise, and core exercises to strengthen that area of the body, you will begin to see your waist measurement come down. When you can move your belt one notch tighter, that will become a constant motivator, showing you that this program is working.

It is also my hope that men reading this book will realize that some of the greatest health risks in our culture, such as type 1 and type 2 diabetes, some forms of cancer, and heart disease, are directly related to abdominal fat. If you carry that extra weight in the midsection into the fourth decade of your life, there is a good chance that within the next ten to fifteen years, you'll be staring some form of disease in the face.

This book is written to give you a thorough understanding of what causes men to gain abdominal fat, and what lifestyle and dietary factors are guaranteed to really take off inches in this area that formerly has been so difficult to reduce. Truly, all things in exercise change, but I believe that this program is something that will stand the test of time because it requires nothing more than going to the grocery and buying everyday foods; walking for 45 minutes to an hour a day, which anybody can do; and doing a series of target abdominal exercises for 15 to 20 minutes four to six times per week, and daily once you've become proficient at them. These core exercises will not only reduce your love handles, but will strengthen your back, alleviating another major problem in our physically inactive culture, low-back pain. This program does not make promises about how much you can get for just "ten minutes a day." I'm more realistic than that. If you are an individual who wants to reduce your waist and strengthen the core area of your body, you just need to be willing to make a commitment for one hour a day. That's all I ask. If you're willing to do that, I can guarantee that you will feel more energetic and see results in your waistline within a month.

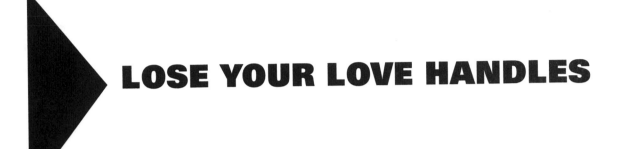

LOSE YOUR LOVE HANDLES

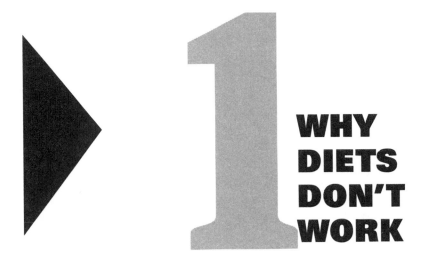

1 ▶ WHY DIETS DON'T WORK

Perhaps you bought this book because you feel that your love handles are a cosmetic problem. You're tired of looking in the mirror and seeing that spare tire that has been developing since you became older or less active. You don't look good in your clothes anymore and feel embarrassed to take off your shirt on a warm day, so you'd like to become leaner and firmer in the waist and abdominal area. But you don't know how. You've already tried some diets and special food plans, but they haven't worked for you. You've "lived hungry," starving yourself to take off pounds, only to put them right back on again. Or you might have joined a gym, but found that the workout you were doing was helping when you first started, but is starting to get diminishing returns. And no matter what machines or weights you've used, nothing really seems to have much effect on those unwanted inches around your waist and in your abdomen. The fat in those areas seems as if it has become permanent, no matter what you do or how hard you work.

You are not alone in your problem. As we enter into the 21st century, America has become one of the fattest societies on earth. Ninety-seven million

3

people, about 55 percent of the adult population, are now considered to be overweight or obese. This number has increased by 8 percent in the last ten years—and continues to grow with no end in sight. Yet we have more diet books, food plans, and health and exercise books to choose from than ever before.

At any given time 25 percent of men—one out of four—are trying to lose weight, and 28 percent are trying to maintain their weight. Much of the unwanted fat in men is in the abdominal area because this is the classic male fat pattern, especially for those over 40. But according to the American College of Sports Medicine, men who diet gain back 67 percent of lost weight within a year, and the remainder within a five-year period. It is safe to say that people today don't really understand what it takes to win the game of weight loss.

Part of the problem is that there is a huge controversy surrounding the subject of how to take off the pounds—and keep them off. Some books tell you that a high percentage of protein in the diet is the key to losing weight. Others say that you have to cut back on carbohydrates. Still others advise that the best course of action is to count calories, or grams of fat.

If you are one of those men who has tried over and over again to take off that spare tire, and failed, this is the book for you. In my over twenty years of studying state-of-the-art medical research, working with over a thousand top athletes, and countless clients like yourself, I have seen extraordinary results. I have learned what it takes to not only take off the love handles, but to increase your metabolism and decrease your risks for diseases like type 2 diabetes, heart disease, high blood pressure, and cancer. I've also learned that many people fail in their weight loss and fitness goals because of widespread misconceptions about what constitutes being overweight and the importance of exercise and proper diet.

What I am offering you in this book is a simple program that will fit easily into your current lifestyle or exercise routine, or that can serve as the basis for you to make a new start if you have not been exercising for quite a while. While following this program will certainly help you to tone and firm the core abdominal area of your body, I encourage you to combine it with circuit training and other resistance exercises that will help you to tone up the entire body. Research has shown that, as we age, resistance exercises and proper nutrition become key to maintaining our health and longevity.

WHY ARE SO MANY AMERICANS OVERWEIGHT?

To begin learning how to lose your love handles, it is necessary for you to understand why men today gain weight in the first place. Why do we have such an epidemic of fat in America? What are we doing wrong, and how can we correct this trend toward increased obesity?

Ironically, the ability to store fat is a trait humans developed half a million years ago to insure the survival of our species. In fact, if the human body didn't have the ability to store fat, we wouldn't be here today. Our ancient ancestors lived in an environment that was very hostile and had no quick and easy sources of food. Early man needed some kind of mechanism to store energy reserves in the body so that they could do the exhausting work of hunting down large animals, often over great distances, and running down small swift animals. These normal fat stores also acted as a buffer to avoid starvation during times of food scarcity. Our female ancestors had the same body mechanism. They stored fat so that they would have enough energy reserves to gather food over great distances and carry and feed their young during lean times.

Naturally, it makes sense that the older the human being became, the less stamina they would have for hunting or gathering. So the body developed an amazing ability—the older the person got, the more easily he was able to store fat for later use. That is one reason why the love handle pattern becomes more of a problem as we get older, because our body doesn't know we aren't struggling to survive. But that is only a part of the picture.

When we switched to an agricultural society about ten thousand years ago, human beings still had to work awfully hard to produce enough to eat. As our culture became more industrialized, things began to change. In the last two generations, our level of activity has dropped radically as machines have taken over more and more of our physical labor. Instead of spending our days hunting or behind a plow, we all too often sit behind a desk, in the seat of a vehicle, or at an assembly line in a factory.

Our eating habits have changed as well. Whereas we used to eat high-fiber grains, lean protein, and fresh fruits and vegetables, we now consume highly processed, low-fiber diets that are high in fats. Because of the state of our large-scale farming industry, which picks many foods before they are ripe so that they can be shipped to the supermarket over great distances, we end up eating few fresh, ripe fruits and vegetables. And much of our produce is grown in soils that have become so depleted in minerals that we get only limited nutritional value from them.

These two factors, less activity and poorly managed dietary habits, have helped to create today's overweight population.

MYTHS ABOUT WEIGHT LOSS

Myth #1: The fewer calories you eat, the more weight you will lose. Wrong! While eating fewer calories than our metabolism requires can help us to lose weight, there is a point of diminishing returns because our metabolism is genetically designed to slow down when food supplies become scarce. In fact, restricting the diet to less than 1,000 calories per day can *severely* decrease metabolism.

Another important part of the equation is the triggering of fat storage. According to Dr. Allen of the Glycemic Research Institute, anytime you go below 1,200 calories a day in a woman, or 1,650 calories a day in a man, you trigger fat storing enzymes because your body—which, anthropologically, is still reacting as it did in prehistory—thinks there's a famine on and that it must start stocking up on reserves.

My recommendation for men losing weight is a low-glycemic diet of between 1,650 and 2,000 calories per day, preferably divided up into three meals and two or three snacks. Distributing calories and carbohydrate foods throughout the day helps to keep your energy level sustained and to normalize insulin. It is also hard to get the nutrients you need if you are only eating one or two meals per day.

Myth #2: Avoid eating carbohydrates. They are fattening. Again, whether or not a food is a carbohydrate is irrelevant. The key, as we shall see, is in the glycemic index of the carb, how slowly it digests and releases its food energy over a period of time so that it will not be stored as fat.

Myth #3: If you want to lose weight and keep it off in the long run, you do not need to exercise. Books by leading diet gurus tend to discount or underplay the value of exercise. While it is certainly true that you can lose weight through eating a well-designed, low-calorie food plan, studies have shown that people usually gain back a significant amount of the weight lost within the first six months of going off the food plan. Current research shows that making regular exercise and cardio-training a part of your life not only helps you to take off weight faster by increasing your metabolism (your ability to burn fat), it is also the *only way* to keep weight off in the long run.

The American College of Sports Medicine states that exercise is one of the most effective ways of controlling insulin resistance. This has been my experience as well. In my work as a performance enhancement specialist, I have seen phenomenal results along this line.

No low-calorie food plan ever created has really worked in the long run. As soon as you go off the diet, the weight comes right back. Exercise and cardio-training, which helps to increase our lean-muscle to fat ratio and decrease our resistance to insulin—coupled with proper nutrition—is the winning ticket.

Myth #4: Our scale weight tells us how thin we are. We live in a culture that lives and breathes by the scale. My advice to you is throw away the scale![1]

Scale weight tells us little about our actual body composition. It all comes down to what a "pound" of weight loss really is. When you try to lose pounds without exercising, what you are really losing is muscle mass, organ tissue, and water, not fat. When you lose a pound through a low-glycemic diet coupled with proper physical exercise and cardio-training, you are insuring that most of your weight loss will be fat. In other words, you are minimizing the loss of your most metabolically active tissue, lean muscle.

Myth #5: Only thin people are healthy. Body weight is not the primary indicator of health. A person can be thin and very unhealthy because they are a couch potato with a high fat to lean-muscle ratio. Again, weight according to the scale tells us little about the really important health factors, such as our ability to manage insulin and our metabolism. A man who at age 50 is "30 pounds overweight," but makes cardio-training and exercise a part of his daily regimen, may actually have a better overall fitness profile and fewer health risks than another 50-year-old who weighs the same as he did when he was in his mid-20's, but has gained added inches of fat in the love handle area.

INSULIN INSENSITIVITY: THE REAL PROBLEM

Belief in these myths will not help you to lose weight in the long run. Now, I'll tell you what *does* work. With a basic understanding of the way our bodies function, the proper diet, and a willingness to put some effort and time into a basic program of cardio-training and resistance exercise, we can bring our weight under control—and keep it there.

As Covert Bailey said in his book *Fit or Fat,* years ago when we were faced with a gasoline crisis, we all got economy cars because smaller engines needed less gas. Since lean muscle mass burns 90 percent of our calories and fat burns 10 percent, putting on an extra 30 to 50 pounds as we age is like becoming an economy version of ourselves (more fat vs. less lean muscle mass). When the fat burning engine (lean muscle) is small, our bodies will economize (store more fat). What we need are cars with bigger engines (more lean muscle vs. fat and a higher metabolism) so that the calories we consume will be burned away.

How do we achieve this goal? Although most diet and fitness books emphasize counting calories for weight loss, the most effective way to reduce weight is through normalizing the body's ability to manage insulin. The ability to manage insulin is based upon four factors: the glycemic index of the foods we eat (their complexity and the amount of time it takes to digest them), our fat to lean-muscle ratio, the efficiency of our metabolism, and the amount of physical activity we engage in. Most of us, as we get older, develop a higher fat to lean-muscle ratio (smaller engine), which leads to a lower metabolic rate and a condition that is known as insulin resistance.

What is insulin resistance and how does it lead to greater storage of food energy in the fat cells? When we eat a meal, our digestive system converts that food into glucose (blood sugar), which is carried in our bloodstream to the pancreas. When our blood is filtered through the pancreas, it measures the amount of glucose present and responds by secreting the amount of insulin needed to carry this blood sugar across the membranes of our cells. In other words, insulin is the hormone responsible for getting energy, in the form of glucose, into our cells.

When a person becomes overweight (fat), he can become insulin resistant. The reason for this is that his muscle cells, which make up 30 to 50 percent of the body, get out of shape and lose much of their ability to respond to insulin. This leaves a surplus of glucose floating around in the blood, much more than the body needs for its immediate metabolic needs. In turn, this stimulates the pancreas to release even more insulin to do its job of transporting the glucose into some kind of cell. Since the fat cells of an overweight individual are more "receptive" to insulin than their muscle cells, that is where much of the remaining glucose eventually gets deposited. This creates a vicious cycle causing even more weight gain. In other words, the more overweight a person becomes, the more nutrients will be stored as fat.

Our pancreas was not overworked during those years of hunting and farming. One reason for this was that our ancestors ate more complex foods, predominantly more complex carbohydrates, which caused a more stable insulin response resulting in leaner, stronger, healthier bodies. These complex foods, which take longer to digest, included things such as whole grains, legumes, and vegetables; all of which have high fiber content and are low in simple sugars. Science has since discovered the glycemic index, which rates foods according to the speed at which they are digested and converted to energy or stored as fat. Foods with a low-glycemic index are more complex and require burning more calories to digest them. Foods with a high-glycemic index digest quickly and, therefore, if not burned during daily activities, are usually stored as fat cells because the body is genetically programmed to store the food energy that we cannot immediately use.

Carbohydrates stimulate the secretion of insulin more than any other type of food that we ingest. When we eat low-glycemic (complex) carbohydrates, the pancreas doesn't have to work as hard because these carbohydrates take time to digest and more of them get burned as energy rather than stored in the fat cells. When our diet consists mainly of simple carbohydrates, such as white bread, soft drinks, and candy bars, foods that are easily and quickly converted into glucose, the pancreas can become overstimulated. If the latter type of eating pattern goes on over a long period of time, the pancreas can become "exhausted," leading to conditions such as type 2 or type 1 diabetes, hypertension, heart disease, and high cholesterol.

Compared to us, our ancestors, who ate slow-digesting, complex carbohydrates and foods, had a lot more lean muscle and a lot less fat in their bodies. They were also much more active, from the time they got up in the morning to the time they went to bed at night. Our modern diet[2] and sedentary lifestyle tend to decrease the amount of lean muscle that we have in our bodies and increase the amount of fat. That's because a diet based on processed and fast foods makes us insulin resistant, leading to greater storage of food energy in fat cells. Take a 20-year-old man who is 5' 8" tall, weighs 140 pounds, and has only 15 percent fat in his body composition, which is a healthy amount of body fat for the average man. By the time this man reaches the age of 30, his scale weight might be the same, but he now has 20 percent body fat because his more demanding workweek and lifestyle have caused him to gradually become less physically active and to eat more fast foods. He may not have put on any extra pounds. But, because fat burns fewer calories than muscle, he is setting himself up for more weight gain, greater insulin resistance, and possibly some serious health risks in later life due to a slower metabolism (less lean muscle to burn calories). An important point to keep in mind is that it is not aging itself that causes a rise in the percentage of body fat, but our decreasing level of activity and the foods that we eat as we grow older. A man can have a healthy body-fat to lean-muscle ratio at any age if he is willing to keep his body fit.

LONG-TERM STRESS CAN CAUSE INSULIN RESISTANCE

Another little-known cause of insulin resistance is long-term stress and what is known as the "stress response." Under normal circumstances, the stress response is a good thing and part of our biological repertoire of survival mechanisms. When we face a stressful situation, our level of the hormones adrenalin and cortisol rise, telling the body to mobilize carbohydrate and fat into the bloodstream to give us a much-needed surge of energy with which to deal with the crisis. The easiest fat to access is abdominal fat, so that is what the body accesses. After the stress response is over, the body returns to balance, but the carbohydrate and fat that has been burned needs to be replenished. When adrenaline levels subside, the remaining cortisol sparks your appetite, making you ravenous. Most people, when refueling after stress, do not reach for a can of tuna or an apple. They want high-carbohydrate foods such as pizza, ice cream, candy bars, or cookies.

It's easy to see that constantly living with stress leads to overeating and an ever-increasing accumulation of abdominal fat. Scientists have discovered that chronically elevated levels of cortisol stimulate fat cells to continually store more fat fuel. That is where the survival mechanism comes into play. In trying to protect itself, the body, which perceives a state of constant "danger," will stock up on the fat it needs to protect itself in times of stress. Of course, this constant cycle—rapid activation of carbohydrate and fat released into the blood stream, fight or flight response, cool down, ravenous eating of carbohydrates (usually in the form of sugar) to restore fat cells—wreaks havoc with the body's insulin response over time.

If you live a life filled with constant stress and want to normalize your insulin response, it is very important to learn how to manage stress through activities such as meditating, exercising, planning ahead, delegating responsibilities, setting priorities, and learning what your limits are.

INSULIN RESISTANCE AND FAT: A SERIOUS HEALTH RISK

That 5 percent body fat you may pick up between the ages of 20 and 30 might not seem so alarming, especially because you still weigh the same. But the issue here is not scale weight, but fat distribution. If you are not adding pounds but are adding inches in your waist line, your health may be at risk. Fat in the love handle area can have serious health consequences.

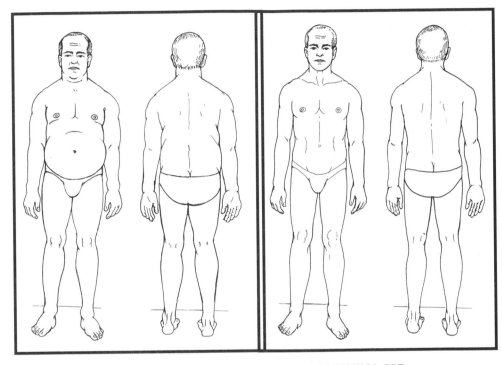

COMPARISON BETWEEN 50-YEAR-OLD MAN WITH ABDOMINAL FAT AND FIT 50-YEAR-OLD MAN.

One of the most dangerous problems associated with abdominal fat, especially in men over the age of 40, is that it lays the groundwork for a person to develop a cluster of symptoms known as "Metabolic Syndrome X," which includes cardiovascular disease and hypertension. The main characteristic of Syndrome X is an increasing resistance to insulin, eventually leading to type 2 diabetes, and, in some cases, to type 1 diabetes. According to the American Diabetes Association, type 2 diabetes and the distribution of fat in the abdominal area are directly related to cardiovascular disease and stroke.

While most people with type 2 diabetes do not have to take insulin, they can develop many uncomfortable symptoms such as frequent urination, general weakness, excessive thirst, predisposition to yeast infections, and poor or slow healing of wounds. Type 2 diabetes accounts for nearly 90 percent of all cases of diabetes, and researchers estimate that 88 to 97 percent of the cases diagnosed in overweight people are the direct result of obesity. What is even more alarming is that this disease, which used to primarily turn up in adults over the age of 40, is now being diagnosed in overweight children and adolescents. According to Dr. Arlan Rosenbloom, professor of pediatrics at the University of Florida in Gainesville, "Children with type 2 can get acutely very ill." It is tragic that our children are also paying with their health for our poor nutrition and sedentary lifestyles.

Dr. Marvin Levin, associate director of the Diabetes and Endocrine Clinic of the American Diabetes Society, agrees with this assessment: "The increase in obesity is one of the leading causes of diabetes. . . . And fifty percent of all diabetics have it and don't know it. That's because the symptoms might not be very prominent yet." High levels of insulin can also accelerate the forming of blood clots, making you more susceptible to strokes and heart attacks.

Dr. Vivien Fonsaka, a professor in the medical school at Tulane University, explains another reason why excess abdominal fat can be a danger:

> . . . this intra-abdominal fat is metabolically very active, and it turns over and releases what I call free fatty acids, which go straight to the liver. Everything within the abdomen drains straight to the liver, where it becomes triglycerides, which is a bad fat that can cause heart disease. Also, in the periphery, the body prefers to burn up fatty acids as fuel rather than glucose. So the glucose gets left behind in the bloodstream and causes its damage that way.

In other words, when we put fat into the core of the body, the abdominal area, we are just asking for trouble because fat stored in the abdominal cavity has a direct pathway to the liver, via an organ called the omentum, where it is converted into "bad fat" and easily circulated throughout the body. When this happens, our LDL—"bad" cholesterol—levels go up and our HDL—"good" cholesterol—levels go down. LDL is the substance that collects in your blood vessels as plaque and clogs them. HDL is the protective type of cholesterol—you can think of it as the garbage collector in your bloodstream. If a small amount of plaque is laid down in the blood vessels and you have enough HDL, it will dissolve the plaque.

It is important to lose your love handles not only to look better but to reduce all of these health risks. The good news, according to Dr. Fonsaka, is that because fat in the abdomen is so metabolically active, it is easier to take off than fat elsewhere in the body. "Physical activity, exercise, and dieting can get rid of that fat fairly quickly. . . . Reduction in the waist-to-hip ratio is a marker for removing the risk of type 2 diabetes." In my experience, doing the *right kind* of exercise is important to lose weight in the abdominal area.

Many other illnesses can be traced to being overweight or obese. The *American Family Physician* reports that one-third of all cases of high blood pressure are associated with obesity, and that obese individuals are 50 percent more likely to have elevated blood cholesterol levels. This journal also states that overweight men are more likely to die of prostate cancers than nonobese men.

According to Dr. Allen at the Glycemic Research Institute, obesity is also related to the increase of many hormonal cancers, such as breast cancer. One reason is that hormones are created and circulate through the fat cells. The more fat cells a person has, and the larger they are, the more chance of the hormones getting out of control and creating hormone-sensitive cancers.

According to new research that Dr. Allen has published in *Women's Fitness* magazine, an obesity-related substance, prostaglanden E2, is directly related to many serious diseases. Overweight or obese people have much higher levels of prostaglanden E2 in their bodies than people of normal weight. High levels of prostaglanden E2 have been linked to both type 1 and type 2 diabetes, hypoglycemia, cancer (particularly colon cancer), and prostate cancer. Dr. Allen's research has also shown that reducing body fat through exercise and proper diet significantly decreases the level of prostaglanden E2 in the body.

The *Journal of the American Medical Association* reports that obesity-related medical conditions contribute to 300,000 deaths every year, second only to smoking as a cause of preventable death.

The costs in trying to treat all of these conditions, most of which could be avoided if we used moderate exercise, cardio-training, and proper diet to increase our metabolism, decrease our fat buildup, and prevent muscle loss, is astronomical. According to the National Heart, Lung, and Blood Institute, over $100 billion is spent per year in the United States on obesity-related medical expenses and loss of income. And Shape Up America! tells us that we spend more than $51.6 billion each year on health care costs related to the cardiovascular complications of obesity. Again, these numbers could be dramatically decreased with modifications to diet and activity level.

THE ROLE OF METABOLISM

One of the first things you must consider when creating a plan to lose your love handles is your metabolic rate. Metabolism is the sum total of all the physical and chemical changes that take place within the body. It includes the transformation of food into energy, the formation of hormones and enzymes, the growth of bone and muscle tissue, and the destruction of body tissue. Our basal metabolic rate, BMR, accounts for approximately 70 percent of our total daily energy expenditure. The energy required to digest and absorb food makes up 5 to 10 percent of our daily energy output, and the energy expended in physical activity utilizes an additional 20 to 30 percent.

The basal metabolic rate represents our basic energy requirements. The most common way to express BMR is in calories per unit of body weight. You can calculate your own RMR (resting metabolic rate) but should have a physician measure your BMR under three sets of circumstances: (1) If you are suddenly gaining weight for no discernable reason, (2) if you are working hard to diet and exercise but can't seem to lose weight, or (3) if you have been yo-yoing up and down weightwise on a variety of different types of diets (in which case, you may have done serious damage to your metabolism). For most readers, however, it will be sufficient to calculate your BMR using the following formula: your weight in kilograms (pounds divided by 2.2) multiplied by 1 calorie multiplied by the number of hours in the day.

If you are an adult male weighing 154 pounds, your basic energy requirements would be 1,880 calories per day.

$$154 / 2.2 = 70 \text{ kg}$$
$$70 \text{ kg X 1 calorie} = 70 \text{ C/hour}$$
$$70 \text{ C X 24 hours} = 1,880 \text{ C per day}$$

However, this figure does not represent the amount of calories you need each day to maintain your current body weight. Because you sit, stand, digest your food, walk, and do other activities that increase your metabolic rate above your BMR—and sleep at night, which lowers it below your BMR—the sum total of all these activities increases your need for calories above the BMR.

Factors such as our genetic makeup, our body type, our body surface area, age, gender, body temperature, and thryroid hormones also influence our BMR.

Usually, the older you become and the more you increase your fat to lean-muscle ratio through inactivity, the slower your metabolism becomes. The good news is that you are not stuck with your metabolic profile. At any age and at any weight, you can change your metabolism through proper diet, cardio-training, and exercise. Many people think that just because they were a marathon runner in their youth, they will be in better physical health in middle to old age after they have stopped being physically active. Wrong. Health depends upon physical activity *in the present.* We can start reaping great benefits from exercise at any age, even if we have never exercised before in our lives. One thing that I tell clients in their 40's, 50's, 60's, and, yes, even their 70's, is that "You are as young as your activity level." In this book I will show you how to determine the level of activity that you need to keep your metabolism efficient.

Recently, E. J. Ourso, a multimillionaire benefactor of Louisiana State University, came to me for help. At 76 years old, he weighed 321 pounds, spent most of his time in a wheelchair, and was taking two insulin shots a day for type 2 diabetes. I put him on an exercise program, but it was so difficult for him to walk that at first he could only use the treadmill for three minutes at a time. After 10 months of eating a low-glycemic diet and doing cardio-training and exercise, he had lost 80 pounds and was able to walk for an hour on the treadmill. Most important, his insulin production had stabilized to the point where he no longer had to take the shots.

Many people will never be able to reach their fantasy weight. But if they follow the guidelines laid down in this book, they will lose body fat, build muscle, improve their aerobic conditioning, normalize their insulin response, decrease their risk of disease, increase their potential longevity, and tone up the abdominal region—an integral part of the body's core area. The key to doing this is through my three-point plan: proper diet, cardiovascular training, and resistance exercises for the core area of the body—the spinal erectors, the abdominal muscles (erectus, transverse, and oblique), the gluteal muscles, the quadriceps, and the hamstrings. If toned and firmed, all of these muscles of the pelvis, which act like a pulley and lever system, will make the love handles disappear.

Reading this book and following its guidelines for nutrition and exercise may be one of the most important things you ever do for yourself. Now, let's get busy and lose those love handles.

CHAPTER NOTES

[1] Scale weight *is* useful if you are involved in intense physical activity and want to use it as a means to check your body's level of hydration. For example, during the practice season, football players and other professional athletes weigh in during the morning and weigh out in the afternoon to see how many pounds of water they have lost during the day.

[2] According to *Webster's Dictionary, diet* is the amount and types of foods we eat to sustain life. In modern life, the word *diet* has become a term we use when we talk about losing weight. Unless specifically indicated, when we use the word *diet*, we are using it more in terms of food plans or healthy nutritional requirements.

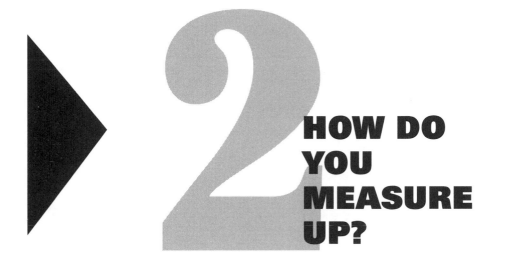

2 HOW DO YOU MEASURE UP?

How much of a risk factor does your fat represent? Are you a ticking time bomb, healthwise? Or are you just starting to put on abdominal fat? In other words, maybe all you need is a good wake-up call to slim and strengthen that core area of your body to help avoid problems in the future. It is never too late to identify the problem, or too early to take steps to prolong the quality and length of your life.

Because there are many conflicting ideas about the definition of being overweight, we aren't going to use weight in pounds to determine health risk. We are going to use two tools—Body Mass Index (BMI) and waist circumference—to evaluate where you stand. There is overwhelming, state-of-the-art medical evidence that says that these criteria are good indicators of fitness, ability to manage insulin, and health risks. These two measurements are used as evaluation tools by medical practitioners, trainers, and major health organizations such as the American Medical Association. I myself have used them for the past decade to help top athletes and ordinary men of all ages to determine their baseline and then to measure their achievements as they reduce fat and increase health and performance.

17

For example, Lomas Brown, who is an NFL player on the offensive line for the New York Giants, came to me when he was having problems with his knee joints. The NFL is always looking for bigger, stronger, and faster linemen. For this reason, many of the men who play this position have enormous BMIs and the attendant health risks because they also have a high percentage of body fat to match their huge size. Lomas came to me initially to get his weight down because of his joint problem, but I discovered that his BMI and his body fat composition were much too high. For this reason, I put him on my three-point program (nutrition, aerobic training, and core exercises), along with his football-specific training, to decrease both his weight and his body fat. At this writing, he's one of the lightest left tackles in football, yet he's at the top of his game after 17 years. I have helped him to convert his smaller size to greater power, which will extend his career—and his life when his career is over.

BODY MASS INDEX: HOW WE MEASURE IT AND WHAT IT TELLS US

Even though Body Mass Index is not infallible, it has become a universal standard for evaluating obesity. Your BMI is your weight in kilograms divided by your height in meters squared. Rather than making you do the math to convert pounds to kilograms and feet and inches to meters, we've done the work for you. You can look up your BMI in Table 2. The numbers moving horizontally across the top column of this table represent weight in pounds. The numbers listed vertically in the far left column represent height in feet and inches. If you find your weight on the horizontal axis, and your height on the vertical axis, your BMI will be at the point where both figures intersect.

	120	130	140	150	160	170	180	190	200	210	220	230	240	250	260	270	280	290	300
5'3"	21	23	25	27	28	30	32	34	36	37	39	41	43	44	46	48	50	51	53
5'4"	21	22	24	26	28	29	31	33	34	36	38	40	41	43	45	46	48	50	52
5'5"	20	22	23	25	27	28	30	32	33	35	37	38	40	42	43	45	47	48	50
5'6"	19	21	23	24	26	27	29	31	32	34	36	37	39	40	42	44	45	47	49
5'7"	19	20	22	24	25	27	28	30	31	33	35	36	38	39	41	42	44	46	47
5'8"	18	20	21	23	24	26	27	29	30	32	34	35	37	38	40	41	43	44	46
5'9"	18	19	21	22	24	25	27	28	30	31	33	34	36	37	38	40	41	43	44
5'10"	17	19	20	22	23	24	26	27	29	30	32	33	35	36	37	39	40	42	43
5'11"	17	18	20	21	22	24	25	27	28	29	31	32	34	35	36	38	39	41	42
6'0"	16	18	19	20	22	23	24	26	27	29	30	31	33	34	35	37	38	39	41
6'1"	16	17	19	20	21	22	24	25	26	28	29	30	32	33	34	36	37	38	40
6'2"	15	17	18	19	21	22	23	24	26	27	28	30	31	32	33	35	36	37	39
6'3"	15	16	18	19	20	21	23	24	25	26	28	29	30	31	33	34	35	36	38
6'4"	15	16	17	18	20	21	22	23	24	26	27	28	29	30	32	33	34	35	37
6'5"	14	15	17	18	19	20	21	23	24	25	26	27	29	30	31	32	33	34	36
6'6"	14	15	16	17	19	20	21	22	23	24	25	27	28	29	30	31	32	34	35

TABLE 2: CALCULATING YOUR BMI

WHAT YOUR BMI MEANS

- A BMI below 20. Unless you are an athlete, a BMI this lean could mean that you are too thin and are possibly compromising your immune system.
- A BMI between 20 and 22 is associated with living the longest and having the lowest incidence of serious illness.
- A BMI between 22 and 25 is still within the acceptable range and is associated with good health.
- If your BMI is between 25 and 30, you are entering the zone where there are serious health risks. A BMI this high puts you at risk for developing type 2 diabetes, heart disease, some cancers, and stroke. You should lower your weight through diet, cardio-training, and exercise.
- If your BMI is over 30, you are definitely putting yourself at risk for all the diseases mentioned above.

According to a study published in the *New England Journal of Medicine*, your life span may decrease significantly if your BMI reaches 25 and may go down even more sharply if your BMI is over 30. A whopping 59 percent of American men now have BMIs over 25.

A study that looked into the health care costs of 17,118 members of the Kaiser Permanente Program of Northern California discovered that the health care expenses for those with a BMI greater than 35 were *twice as much* as those with a BMI between 20 and 25. The greatest increases in spending were, not surprisingly, for drugs used to treat diabetes, hypertension, and cardiovascular disease. Obese individuals also spent more on medications to treat pain, depression, respiratory illness, and ulcers.

Remember, the BMI is not infallible. That is why I am giving you other self-evaluation tools to use along with it. The BMI will not correctly reflect the health of weight lifters, professional athletes, and other individuals who have a greater BMI due to elevated muscle mass rather than excess fat. A 6' 2" athlete who weighs 225 pounds might have a BMI of 27 or 28, which seems too high. Yet that person might have only 4 percent body fat. In order to evaluate where you stand, body compositionwise and healthwise, you always need more than one criteria.

WAIST CIRCUMFERENCE

The circumference of the waist is, hands down, the most important and reliable indicator of health risks. An article in the *Canadian Journal of Diabetes Care* showed that an increase in the waist was always a clear indicator that fat was collecting in the abdominal area, especially in men between the ages of 40 and 60 years of age.

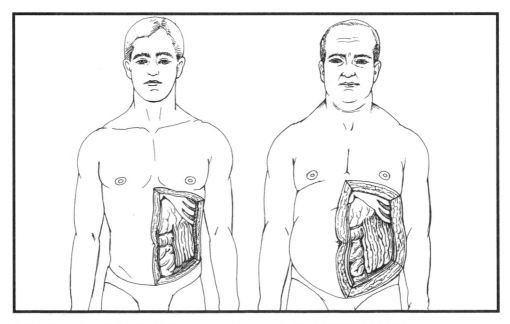

HOW FAT COLLECTS IN THE ABDOMINAL AREA AS AGE INCREASES

In one seven-year study, even though the subjects' scale weight and BMI remained the same, there was a marked increase in the waist measurement accompanied by a 30 percent increase in abdominal fat. The subjects also became more insulin resistant over this time period, making them more likely to store glucose in the fat cells in the abdominal area, which accounted for the expanding waistlines. In other words, they were becoming prime candidates for type 2 diabetes.

Other studies have borne this out. According to Dr. J. Pervis Milnor III et al. in the book *It Can Break Your Heart: What You and Your Doctor Should Know About Solving Your Weight Problem,* when a man's waist circumference exceeds 40 inches, he is not only at greater risk for developing type 2 diabetes, but higher cholesterol levels, leading to coronary disease. Health risks are especially high when both waist size and BMI exceed the standard levels.

▶ If you want to accurately measure your waist circumference, use a tape to measure at the level of the last rib, known as the "floating rib" because it does not connect to the sternum, but to the rib above it.

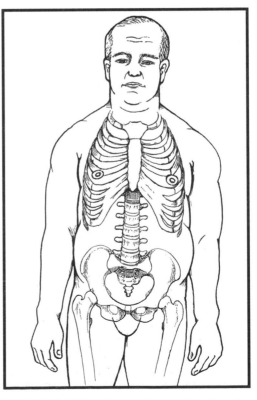

WHERE TO MEASURE YOUR WAIST

A recent study done by the National Heart, Lung, and Blood Institute, rated men's risk for type 2 diabetes, hypertension, and cardio disease according to the following criteria:

- If you have a BMI of 25.5 to 29.9 and a waist of 40 inches, you are considered overweight and you are in an increased risk category. If your BMI remains the same, but your waist exceeds 40 inches, your risk for these diseases falls into the very high category.
- If you have a BMI of 30 to 34.9, you are considered to suffer from Class I Obesity. If your waist is 40 inches, your health risks are high. If your waist exceeds 40 inches, your risks for type 2 diabetes, hypertension, and cardiovascular disease becomes very high.
- If your BMI is between 35 and 39.9 and you have a waist of 40 inches or more, you are diagnosed with Class II Obesity and your health risks are very high.

A recent study funded by the National Cancer Institute, the National Heart, Lung, and Blood Institute, and the American Cancer Society found that men who were overweight were more likely to have erectile dysfunction than their slimmer counterparts. Men with a waistline of 42 inches or more were more than twice as likely to have this problem, even after adjusting for risk factors such as age, smoking, and hypertension. This study also showed that men who were inactive were more prone to erectile dysfunction than men who exercised for at least 30 minutes a day.

The good news is that it is never too late to lose fat in the waist area and to bring that measurement down.

Of course, a waist circumference of 40 inches and above is not an absolute value. A man who is 6' 2" tall, or someone who is big boned, would naturally have a bit more leeway than a man who is 5' 8" tall, or of a smaller bone structure. The taller, bigger man could actually have a larger waist measurement, but not yet be considered in a risk category. On the other hand, an ectomorph body type (tall and extremely thin) could likely be at risk even if his waist measurement were somewhat smaller than 40 inches. For most of us, the average is a good indication that we should seriously consider eating a better diet and exercising to reduce that part of the body.

MEASURING YOUR RATIO OF FAT TO LEAN-MUSCLE

Another measurement that may help in giving you a full picture of your body composition is the ratio of fat to lean-muscle. As we get older and more inactive, most of us gain more body fat relative to the amount of lean muscle we carry. This leads to a slower metabolic rate, a decreased ability to manage insulin, and a greater vulnerability to certain health risks. Having a proper fat to lean-muscle ratio is important because muscle burns 90 percent of our calories. The more muscle mass you have, the more calories you burn, even in a resting state. A good target goal for most men is to aim for having between 8 and 16 percent body fat.

What do we mean when we talk about lean body weight as opposed to fat body weight? Lean body weight includes the muscles, bones, ligaments and tendons, tissues and water of our bodies. Fat body weight is how much fat we carry. As we have so clearly seen, standing on a scale and seeing how much we weigh is useless when it comes to accurately measuring our body composition. This is because a volume of fat weighs about half as much as an equal volume of muscle. Two people can actually be the same height and the same weight, but look very different from one another. While one man looks very thin and muscular, the other may look soft and pudgy because he has a much higher percent of fat in his body composition.

There are several methods used to determine your fat to lean-muscle ratio. Keep in mind, however, that there is always a range of error in the less expensive tests.

Hydrostatic Weighing: Although the most expensive (costing between $100 and $150), this method is currently considered the "gold standard" of body composition analysis. Hydrostatic measurements are based on the assumption that density and specific gravity of lean tissue is greater than that of fat tissue. For this reason, lean tissue should sink in water and fat tissue should float. By comparing a test subject's mass measured while under water with his mass measured while out of the water, a fairly accurate fat to lean-muscle ratio can be calculated.

You can usually find a facility for doing hydrostatic weighing at a local university, hospital wellness center, college, health club, or fitness center that is set up to do this measurement for the public. You can either call these facilities in your area to see if they offer hydrostatic weighing or ask your doctor for a recommendation.

Skin Fold Measurement with a caliper: This is the second most common method of ascertaining your fat to lean-muscle ratio. It involves measuring your subcutaneous fat, the fat under your skin, by using a measuring device such as a caliper. One of the pluses of this method is that it has been around for a long time and is readily available to the public through hospitals, physical therapy centers, health clubs, schools, universities, exercise physiologists, dietitians, and Jazzercise instructors. It is also very reasonably priced, costing between $5 to $15. This test has a plus or minus 6 percent error rate.

Anthropometric Measurement: This is another quick, easy, and inexpensive method to estimate body composition. This test is based on the assumption that body fat is distributed at various sites on the body such as the neck, wrist, and waist. Muscle tissue, on the other hand, is usually located at locations such as the biceps, forearm, and calf. A person's weight, height, girth size, and the ratios of various site comparisons are used to calculate the percent of body fat present. You can probably get this test done at many of the same locations where you can get the skin fold measurement performed. This test has a plus or minus 5 percent rate of error. If you wish to perform this measurement yourself, follow the steps below.

▶ **ANTHROPOMETRIC MEASUREMENT**

1. Using a regular tape measure, determine the following measurements in inches:

Measure at the navel   Waist: _____

Measure in front of the bones where the wrist bends   Wrist: _____

2. Subtract the wrist from the waist measurement   _____

3. Write down your weight in pounds   _____

4. Look up your percent body fat using the table below by using the number you got in step 2 (horizontal value in table) and your body weight (vertical value in table).

Example: Waist = 36.0 inches   Estimated body composition = 22% (% fat

Wrist =   6.5 inches   to lean-muscle)

29.5 inches

Weight = 170 lbs.

Weight	22	22½	23	23½	24	24½	25	25½	26	26½	27	27½	28	28½	29	29½	30	30½	31	31½	32	32½	33	33½	34	34½	35
130	3	5	7	9	11	12	14	16	18	20	21	23	25	27	28	30	32	34	36	37	39	41	43	44	46	46	50
135	3	5	7	8	10	12	13	15	17	19	20	22	24	26	27	29	31	32	34	36	38	39	41	43	44	46	48
140	3	5	6	8	10	11	13	15	16	18	19	21	23	24	26	28	29	31	33	34	36	38	39	41	43	44	46
145	3	4	6	7	9	11	12	14	15	17	18	20	22	23	25	27	28	30	31	33	35	36	38	39	41	43	44
150	2	4	6	7	9	10	12	13	15	16	17	19	21	23	24	26	27	29	30	32	34	35	36	38	40	41	43
155	2	4	5	7	8	10	11	13	14	16	17	19	20	22	23	25	26	28	29	31	33	34	35	37	38	40	41
160	2	4	5	6	8	9	11	12	14	15	16	18	19	21	22	24	25	27	28	30	31	33	34	35	37	38	40
165	2	3	5	6	8	9	10	12	13	15	15	17	19	20	22	23	24	26	27	29	30	31	33	34	36	37	38
170	2	3	4	6	7	9	10	11	13	14	15	17	18	19	21	22	24	25	26	28	29	30	32	33	34	36	37
175	2	3	4	6	7	8	10	11	12	14	14	16	17	19	20	22	23	24	25	27	29	29	31	32	33	35	36
180		3	4	5	7	8	9	10	12	13	14	16	17	18	19	21	22	23	25	26	28	28	30	31	32	34	35
185		2	4	5	6	8	9	10	11	13	13	15	16	18	19	21	21	23	24	25	27	28	29	30	31	33	34
190		2	4	5	6	7	9	10	11	12	13	15	16	17	18	20	21	22	23	24	26	27	28	29	30	32	33
195		2	3	4	6	7	8	9	10	12	12	14	15	16	18	19	20	21	22	24	25	26	27	28	29	31	32
200		2	3	4	6	7	8	9	10	11	12	14	15	16	17	19	19	21	22	23	24	26	26	28	28	30	31
205		2	3	4	5	6	8	9	9	11	12	13	14	15	17	18	19	20	21	22	23	25	26	27	27	29	30
210		2	3	4	5	6	7	8	9	11	11	13	14	15	16	18	18	19	21	22	23	25	25	26	26	28	29
215			3	4	5	6	7	8	9	10	11	12	13	14	16	17	18	19	20	21	22	24	24	26	26	28	29
220			2	4	4	6	7	8	9	10	11	12	13	14	15	17	17	18	19	20	21	23	24	25	25	27	28
225			2	3	4	6	7	8	8	10	10	12	13	13	15	16	17	18	19	20	21	23	23	25	24	26	27
230			2	3	4	5	6	7	8	9	10	11	12	13	14	16	16	17	18	19	20	22	22	24	23	25	26
235			2	3	4	5	6	7	8	9	10	11	12	13	14	15	16	17	18	19	20	22	22	23	23	25	26
240			2	3	4	5	6	7	8	9	9	11	12	13	13	15	16	17	17	18	20	21	21	23	22	24	25
245			2	3	4	5	6	7	8	9	9	10	11	13	13	15	16	16	17	18	19	21	21	22	22	24	25
250			2	3	4	5	6	6	7	8	9	10	11	13	13	14	15	16	17	18	19	20	20	21	22	23	24
255			2	3	3	4	5	6	7	8	9	10	11	12	13	14	15	15	16	17	18	20	20	21	21	23	24
260			2	2	3	4	5	6	7	8	9	10	10	11	12	13	14	15	16	17	18	19	19	20	21	22	23

Bioelectrical Impedance: Safe, accurate, and convenient, biolectrical impedance is based upon the fact that the body's lean tissue is much more conductive than fat due to its higher water content. To perform this test, a health care professional attaches a bioimpedance meter to the body, at the extremities, and uses a small 500–800 microamp, 50 kilohertz signal to measure the body's ability to conduct this current. The more lean tissue present in the body, the greater the conductive potential, measured in ohms.

This machine is dependent on your level of hydration, so if you have just finished a workout or drunk a lot of coffee or alcohol, activities that have dehydrating effects, the test will not be accurate. There is a 5 to 6 percent margin of error compared to the results of the hydrostatic weighing test.

When deciding how much of a health threat your fat to lean-muscle ratio is, it is always important to keep the big picture in mind. While the body fat of a normal man should usually not drop below 8 percent, elite male athletes may have a fat percentage as low as 3 percent in their overall body composition.

Do keep in mind, however, that while following the program in this book will help you to lose overall body fat, it is primarily designed to help you lose and firm the waist and abdominal region—the core area of the body.

EVALUATING YOUR HEALTH

While it's not absolutely necessary to the success of this program, there are certain general health-evaluation tests that a person should have done periodically by his family doctor. I asked my personal physician, Dr. Kathleen Wilson, what regular checkups and tests she would recommend for men, based on their age. Dr. Wilson is an internist for the prestigious Ochsner Clinic in New Orleans and, for many years, was the personal physician of generals and other important personnel in the U.S. Air Force.

As Dr. Wilson points out, any periodic test a person should receive depends upon their personal health profile and family history. Not all people need all tests at every interval. On average, however, she has found that people in the 20- to 40-year-old age group should have:

■ A lipid profile, a test that measures HDL (good cholesterol) and LDL (bad cholesterol) every 5 to 10 years.

- A fasting glucose test for blood sugar every 5 years to see if they have diabetes or a tendency toward diabetes. (The term *fasting glucose* refers to the fact that your doctor will ask you not to eat after midnight before the morning of the test.)
- A blood pressure check every 2 to 5 years if blood pressure is normal.
- A physical every 2 to 3 years.

If you are overweight, you should also have a thyroid stimulating hormone (TSH) test to measure whether your thyroid might be underactive. This test is done for someone with high cholesterol because high cholesterol can be a sign of an underactive thyroid.

People's health maintenance needs begin to change in the 40- to 60-year-old age group. During these decades, a person should have:

- A lipid profile every 5 years.
- A fasting glucose test every 5 years.
- A blood pressure check every 2 years, if the blood pressure is normal.
- A physical every 2 years.

At age 50, it is routine to start screening for two kinds of cancers: prostate and colon. Unless a person has high blood pressure, he does not need to have a baseline EKG until he reaches 50.

After a person has reached the age of 60, the disease burden in the population is high enough that tests need to be person specific depending upon your individual health profile. Sixty is also the age when you may consider taking your first stress test, unless you already have symptoms of heart disease, in which case you should take this test when these symptoms appear.

Getting these tests done can help to shed even more light on your overall health profile and how you might use my wellness program to benefit you the most. The more you know about the present state of your body, the more effectively you can follow the food plan, cardio-train, and exercise to achieve your goals. Remember, before embarking on this or any other nutrition and exercise program, it is wise to check with your personal physician or health care professional.

INTRODUCING THE SIX CASE STUDIES: HOW THEY MEASURED UP

When I decided to write this book, I realized that the best way to demonstrate how this program works (and how noticeable benefits could be achieve in as little as 30 days), was to ask six test subjects to follow the program for one month. Interestingly, the participants in the program were so happy with their results, and found my wellness program so comfortable to follow, that they decided to make it a part of their lifestyle. For this reason, I was fortunate to also be able to remeasure them at the 8-week interval and then again at the 12-week interval.

Below are the initial measurements of the six participants showing their initial weight, waist measurement, BMI, and body fat percent at the onset of the program.

Name:	Age:	Height:	Weight:	Waist:	BMI:	Body Fat %:
Bob	37	6' ½"	206 lbs.	37 in.	27.4	25.8%
Don	38	6' 3"	224 lbs.	39.5 in.	28.6	20.6%
Stan	46	6' 1"	231 lbs.	40.5 in.	27.3	30.0%
Dorian	46	5' 10"	194 lbs.	38.5 in.	27.6	24.7%
Jerry	45	6' 2"	266 lbs.	46.25 in.	34.2	21.0%
Rob	44	5'11"	197.5 lbs.	39.25 in.	27.7	22.9%

FIGURE 2.4: ABDOMINAL PROTOCOL—NOVEMBER 21, 1999

All of these men had different reasons for wanting to be a part of this program. Jerry is a police captain who puts in a lot of hours at work and is on call 24 hours a day. When I approached him about the possibility of being one of the test subjects, he immediately agreed because of "the confidence I have in you." With a waist of 46.25, a BMI of 34.2, and a body fat level of 21 percent, Jerry was in the highest risk group for health problems such as type 2 diabetes, heart disease, some cancers, and stroke.

Dorian is a professional real estate broker who runs his own office and describes his work as "highly stressful." When I first suggested to him that he volunteer for the 30-day program, he was a bit hesitant. But his hesitancy soon changed to enthusiasm when he saw the results he was getting. Dorian's waist initially measured 38.5 inches, his BMI was 27.6, and his body fat percentage was 24.7. These figures also represented possible health risks.

Stan is a professional teaching golf pro. Stan decided to participate in this program because "I'd gotten so out of shape that I really was uncomfortable, and I felt like it was hurting my golf game and my performance. I decided it was time to try to shape up and get healthy again." While Stan admitted that he knew he was never going to be in the shape he was in when he was in his 20's, he believed he could improve his health and fitness to a very great degree. He also has the dream of playing golf on the senior tour, and realizes that he has to get into a lot better shape to do that. The day Stan shared these goals with me, I told him about the program and got him started. On November 21, the official start date of the program, Stan's waist measurement was 38.5, his BMI 27.3, and his fat percentage 20.9. Stan had actually begun this program about two months before the other participants, so by the November date he had already lost 2 inches in the waist and his percentage of body fat had dropped a whopping 10 points!

Bob is a police officer. Although he has been exercising, running, and lifting weights off and on for the last 15 years, he felt that he wasn't getting the results he needed from his workout. He had hit a plateau and couldn't seem to move off it. With a waist of 37, a BMI of 27.4, and a body fat percentage of 25.8, Bob started with better statistics than many of the guys in the test group, but he was still in the health risk category. When I told him about the 30-day study and asked if he would like to be a participant, he jumped at the chance.

Rob is also a police officer. He had already participated in one 30-day program that I had designed to help people reach a target heart rate. He wasn't a member of a gym at the time of the study, but when I approached him, he was eager to be one of the test subjects. He said he had heard some of the guys talking about the new program, and that they were very enthusiastic about trying it. At the start of the study, Rob's waist was 39.25, his BMI was 27.7, and his body fat percentage was 22.9. Again, he wasn't in the highest risk group, but his health was certainly at risk.

Don, a former football player at Tulane University, is a junior high school teacher and a football coach for young boys. When I ran into him at a school function, he was looking for a new workout program. He asked, "Mackie, can you write me a prescription to help me reduce body fat and increase muscle tone?" I told him that it just so happened that I was about to start a program, and that he might find some benefits in it. Don's waist was 39.5 inches, his BMI was 28.6, and his percent body fat percentage was 20.6. At 6' 3", Don was the tallest guy in the test group, so one might argue that this should be taken into account when assessing his risk of disease. Maybe it would be normal for some of Don's measurements to be a couple of inches above the norm. Yet that all-important waist measurement of his was the second highest in the group, indicating that he carried a lot of fat in the abdominal area. This, as we have seen, is a red flag and a problem that only gets worse as a person ages. It is also important to note that, at age 38, Don is also the *youngest* man in the group, which means that he is putting on a significant amount of inches in the waist before he has even reached his high-risk forties.

I deliberately decided to run this study during the most stressful 30 days of the year, between Thanksgiving and the Christmas and Hanukkah season. As we shall see, these men lost a considerable amount of weight, body fat, and inches during that time. If they could do this program when stress levels were high, spare time was limited, and there were plenty of tempting holiday meals and parties, *anyone can do it.* And the best news of all is that the men found the program relatively easy to follow. In fact, it gave them so many psychological and physical benefits, that they wanted to make it a permanent part of their lifestyle.

To help you get started, here is a chart in which you can record your baseline measurements and assess your progress at monthly intervals. Measuring your body composition, your fat to lean-muscle ratio, is optional. If you do decide to get this measurement taken, however, keep in mind that it is not necessary to do so every month. Twelve-week intervals will be sufficient. You can record your measurements in the weekly Progress Chart I have included below. (Figure 2.5)

	Weight:	Waist:	BMI:	% Body Fat (optional):
Day 1:				
Week 4:				
Week 8:				
Week 12:				*
Week 16:				
Week 20:				
Week 24:				*

FIGURE 2.5: YOUR PROGRESS CHART

Remember that making any new program a part of your routine will involve a little adjustment in the beginning. Each of the six test subjects said that it took him about a week or so of eating low-glycemic foods, practicing the cardio-walking, and doing the resistance exercises to really hit his stride and make the program a part of his routine. Just remember, however, that consistency is the key to making this program work—and consistency is what will help you watch those love handles melt away.

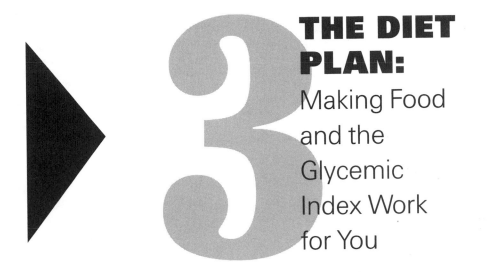

3

THE DIET PLAN:

Making Food and the Glycemic Index Work for You

The first part of my 3-point plan for getting rid of abdominal fat is learning what strategies go into creating a healthy diet—and the best way to put them all together. In spite of all the diet books and fads that are on the market, many people really have little or no idea about how to take off weight and *keep it off*. I know, because I've spent years watching people unsuccessfully try to diet and take off inches. Most people believe that you have to live hungry, or eat exotic health foods, or avoid carbohydrates or fats altogether. While these ideas may work in the short run, they fail in the long run because of one very basic scientific fact: They do not deal with the real problem, which is not losing weight, but retraining your sluggish metabolism and your insulin resistance, the basic mechanisms that cause your body to store unhealthy amounts of fat.

▶ **LEARNING TO EAT FOR SUCCESS**
INVOLVES FOUR BASIC STRATEGIES:

- ◆ Adopting some easy-to-follow strategies, "Mackie's Dietary Dos and Don'ts."
- ◆ Understanding the Glycemic Index and using it to choose your optimum foods.
- ◆ Learning what percentages of fat, carbohydrates, and protein should be a part of your daily diet—and why.
- ◆ Estimating your caloric requirements and using them to follow my basic meal plans.

The good news is that, unlike most diets, which are designed around depriving yourself of calories, you will never feel hungry on my program. The test subjects who followed my food plan felt satisfied with the types and amounts of food I recommended, and they also felt that they had many appetizing and interesting choices. All of them told me that it was so easy to stay on my low-glycemic food plan that they intended to continue to make it a permanent part of their lifestyle.

DIETARY DOS AND DON'TS

One of the most important things to understand about losing inches in the love handle area is that eating a healthy diet involves changing some of your habits; habits having to do with when you eat, how often you eat, and what you eat. Do you skip breakfast, the most important meal of the day, and then grab a high-glycemic, fast-food lunch? Do you save up all your calories for one big meal at the end of the day, causing your blood sugar to shoot up right before you go to bed so that your body stores this energy as fat while you sleep? Do too many of your meals consist of pizza, sugars, and fried foods?

If training your insulin to help get rid of abdominal fat is your goal, here are some basic strategies to help you succeed.

Mackie's Dietary Dos
Only eat glycemically acceptable foods. According to Dr. Ann de Wees Allen, N.D., Director of Research and Development for the Glycemic Research Institute in Washington, D.C. (www.anndeweesallen.com), figuring out which foods are low-glycemic and which are not is not something you can do using common sense. For example, one of our most popular diet foods, rice cakes, has a very high glycemic index. It actually makes us gain weight! Ice cream, one of the foods that we think of as fattening, has a low

glycemic index. Why? Because ice cream contains protein. (On pages 40–51 I'll provide you with a list of low-glycemic and high-glycemic foods.)

Eat 3 meals and 2 to 3 snacks per day. I suggest 7:00 A.M., 9:30 A.M., noon, 3 P.M., 6:30 P.M., 8:00 P.M., but you can adjust these times, depending upon your schedule. For example, if you are a night owl who only needs five hours' sleep and regularly goes to bed at 2:00 A.M. and wakes up at 7:00 A.M., you would need to space these meals out a bit further. Distributing calories and carbohydrate foods throughout the day helps keep your energy level sustained. Waiting until your blood sugar is low and you are starving does nothing for fat loss. Instead, your body will adapt to what it perceives as a starvation regime, and use less energy, making weight loss even harder. A good rule of thumb is to try not to go longer than 4 to 5 hours between meals. A list of sample meals and low-fat snacks are included in this chapter.

Drink adequate fluids. On days that you exercise, you should drink two-thirds of your body weight in ounces of nonsugar fluid—preferably water. On nonexercise days, you should drink about one-half of your body weight in ounces. So, if you weigh 160 pounds, on a nonexercise day you should drink 80 ounces of water or other fluids (there are 128 ounces in a gallon), or about 3 quarts. When you are working out, you should try to drink close to one gallon of fluids. These are the healthy minimums, but it could benefit you to drink a bit more. At first, frequency of urination will increase, but your body will adjust to the greater water intake over time.

Whether you are an athletic person or just lead an active lifestyle, proper hydration is an important ingredient for overall good health. If you shortchange your body of its water supply, your ability to operate at peak efficiency will be reduced. When facing a shortage, the kidneys will retain water in order to prevent what they perceive as dehydration. Some hunger signs are actually signals that your body is thirsty. Other signs include body aches, muscle tightness, skin dryness, and sluggishness.

Increase your intake of low-glycemic fruits, vegetables, and whole grains such as apples, yams, whole wheat bread, and oatmeal. These foods are packed with carbohydrates for energy and vitamins and will give you needed fiber and provide you with a feeling of fullness.

Limit your intake of animal fats (red meat, high-fat dairy products, whole eggs). These are high in saturated fats, the kind of fat that clogs your blood vessels.

Eat lean meats, broiled, grilled, or baked. Baste them with olive oil, not butter. Remove the skin from chicken.

Have cold-water fish such as tuna, salmon, and halibut at least twice per week.

Include at least one high-fiber-source food with each meal. You will find these whole-grain breads, cereals, legumes, fresh fruits, and raw vegetables in the section of this chapter entitled "Glycemically Acceptable Foods," pages 40-46.

Oils. Use olive, canola, peanut, or flax oil with vinegar or lemon juice on salads, along with spices, or a dressing from the "Glycemically Acceptable Foods" section of this chapter (pages 40-46).

Eat one good source of vitamin C per day. Citrus, strawberries, tomatoes, and melons are good vitamin C foods.

Have one good source of vitamin A foods three to four times per week. Sweet potato; V8 juice; and dark green, leafy vegetables are good vitamin A foods.

Make soy foods a part of your diet. One of the easiest ways to do this is to use soy powder as a snack, preferably in increments of 20 grams of protein a day. I suggest Personal Edge® Fat Metabolizer Drink Mix, the natural, sugar-free version (1 serving = 2 scoops = 20 grams of protein). Have ½ serving (1 scoop) as your morning snack, and the other ½ serving around 8:00 P.M. in low-fat milk or, if you are lactose intolerant, in unsweetened orange juice, water, or a nonsugar beverage.

Use energy bars as a snack. Many energy bars have a high sugar content, so I suggest a Personal Edge® Soy Energy Bar, an Atkins Advantage Bar, a Met-Rx Protein Plus Bar, or a Worldwide Pure Protein Bar, along with a medium-sized low-glycemic fruit, such as an apple, orange, or pear.

Use Promise or Take Control butter alternatives, or Fleishman's margarine. When dining out, use butter in moderation since it is a saturated fat. Soft butter and stick margarine can elevate trans-fatty acids and potentially increase LDL, bad cholesterol, as well as decreasing HDL, good cholesterol.

Get adequate rest—at least 7 hours per night.

Use wine and hard liquor in moderation. Mix liquor with noncaloric beverages. Never drink after 8:00 P.M.

Take your supplements on schedule. The most important supplements are multivitamins, antioxidants, calcium, magnesium, zinc, and vitamin C. Taking antioxidants is especially important because your body will be producing cancer-causing free radicals as you do the cardio-walking and the resistance exercises. Antioxidants will help in neutralizing these free radicals. As your body gets used to this new level of exercise over time, it will release fewer free radicals, but it is still a good idea to take these supplements.

Seek the advice of a professional. If you feel that you need additional help with healthy eating to fuel fitness and burn off the fat, seek the advice of a professional such as a registered, licensed dietician. A good place to find one is by E-mailing or phoning the American Dietetic Association at www.eatright.org, 1-800-366-1655. This national organization will help you to find a qualified professional in your area. It is important to make sure that someone is both registered *and* licensed. Many people out there who call themselves nutritionists, or who do nutritional counseling in health clubs, are not necessarily qualified to create meal plans that are medically safe, based upon sound principals, and meet your personal needs.

Mackie's Dietary Don'ts

Don't eat simple sugars. The refined sugars found in table sugar, honey, cakes, cookies, soft drinks, and candy need to go—they help fat to stay put. Avoid white breads, white flour, white potatoes, and regular white pastas. Use whole wheat breads, whole wheat pastas, and sweet potatoes instead.

Don't skip meals. Adjust to your daily schedule.

Don't eat after your 8:00 P.M. snack. Your body needs time to digest your food.

Avoid all fried or glycemically unacceptable foods.

Do not go below 1,650 calories per day. If you eat less than this, your body will respond as if there is a famine and will begin to store fat to stock up on reserves.

Understanding the Glycemic Index

Although the Industrial Revolution brought us many technological miracles, giving us tools for preserving, storing, and enhancing foods, in many ways it has been a real setback for the human diet. Unlike our ancestors, who got plenty of fiber and all of the nutrients they needed from the fresh fruits and vegetables, coarsely ground grains, and lean meats that were the staples of their diet, we have become a processed and fast-food culture. The average American diet has made us insulin resistant, causing us to store fat in unhealthy amounts, primarily in the abdominal area.

Dr. Ann de Wees Allen, one of the head researchers for the Glycemic Institute, describes the problem this way.

"If you were to hire some geneticists and say, 'How can we create a society that is going to have real health and medical problems?' you'd be doing exactly what we're doing now, which is to take a species that isn't designed to hold a large amount of body fat, and then start adding fat from a very young age. That's probably the worst thing you can do. And it's reflected in the fact that, in the U.S., we have the fastest growing and highest rate of body fat of any country in the world. And we have the attendant medical problems that match that increased body fat."

Long before the advent of wonder drugs and antibiotics, our grandparents knew that food is the first medicine; the first line of scrimmage for preserving our health. This is still true today. I have found that eating the proper types of food in increments of three meals and two or three snacks a day does wonders for the body because it enables a person to take in food at the rate at which they can use it. What do I mean by the "proper types of food"? In the last two decades, leading-edge scientific research has shown that one of the best tools for eating right is the glycemic index.

The glycemic index is a ranking of foods according to their immediate effect on blood sugar levels. The key is the rate of digestion. Foods that are high-glycemic digest very quickly, causing your blood sugar to soar. If this energy is not used, then it is converted into fat by the liver. Low-glycemic foods are those that digest slowly, releasing their energy over a longer period of time.

Most of the time you would want to minimize the amount of high-glycemic foods in your diet, except under special circumstance. If you are an athlete, a couple of hours before your sports event you would benefit from eating low-glycemic index foods that digest slowly and give you energy and endurance. After the event, or between multiple events, you would benefit from eating high-glycemic foods to help you replenish your energy stores and have greater staying power. Likewise, if you are a day hiker or backpacker about to take a strenuous climb up a mountain with a heavy pack on your back, you would begin with a slow-digesting, low-glycemic breakfast for endurance. You would plan to have a mixed-glycemic lunch and periodically snack throughout the day on high-glycemic nuts, dried fruits, and power bars to restore your energy reserves and keep you going. But if you are going to sit at your desk for the rest of the afternoon, you don't need an explosion of energy, and a high-glycemic lunch, plus a candy bar and a bag of potato chips for a midafternoon snack; these are guaranteed to add to your spare tire.

It is important to remember, however, that these high- and low-glycemic foods lists are meant as a guide. If you include a high-glycemic food in your meal plan once in awhile, it will not harm you. The high glycemic rating of a food can also be neutralized by eating it in combination with other low-glycemic foods. For example, if you eat a ripe banana with some lean protein, it won't cause your blood sugar to soar.

There is no way to logically figure out which foods are high-glycemic and which are not just by looking at them. White potatoes are high-glycemic, but sweet potatoes are not because they are not a member of the potato family, but of the nightshade family. Watermelon is high-glycemic, but honeydew melon is low-glycemic. The glycemic index of pasta goes up the longer you cook it, and that of bananas increases as they ripen. Although rice is generally thought of as a glycemically unacceptable food, short-grain rice has a much higher glycemic rating than long-grain rice.

To make it easy for you, I have included a low-glycemic acceptable foods list, and a high-glycemic unacceptable foods list. If you want further information on the glycemic index and other dietary-related topics, the Glycemic Institute offers some great books that you may order through their Web site at www.glycemic.com or by calling (727) 344-2328. The Glycemic Institute also evaluates some packaged foods and provides a Seal of Approval. (Worldwide Pure Protein Bars, page 45, received this endorsement.) It is always a good idea to read the labels of the foods you buy. For example, on page 59, we give a list of the label names of hidden sugars in packaged and fat-free foods.

GLYCEMICALLY ACCEPTABLE FOODS[1]

Fruit (Fresh)

Apple

Applesauce, unsweetened

Banana, green

Blueberries

Boysenberries

Casaba melon

Cantaloupe

Cherries

Figs, fresh only

Grapes

Grapefruit

Honeydew melon

Kiwi

Lemon

Lime

Mandarin orange

Nectarine

Orange

Peach

Pear

Persimmon

Plantains

Plum

Pomegranate

Raspberries

Strawberries

Tangerines

Jams and Jellies

(low glycemic jams and jellies are those made:)

With low glycemic fruits

Without grape juice

Without high glycemic juice

Without corn syrup or

    added unacceptable sugar

Fruit (Canned)

Libby's Natural Lite

    Pear halves

    Sliced peaches

    Peach halves

    Chunky Mixed Fruits

    Fruit cocktail

Super Giant Juice Pack

    Peaches

    Pears

Mott's Natural Applesauce

White House Natural Plus Applesauce

Pure Unsweetened Fruit Juices

(From fruit only, no added sugar, high fructose corn syrup, grape juice, or pineapple juice—limited to 1/2 cup)

Apple juice

Orange juice

Peach juice

Pear juice

Grapefruit juice

Orange juice with pulp

    Tropicana Grovestand

(Because of the potential of juices to elevate blood sugar, you should limit their consumption. Try mixing 1/2 cup juice with 1/2 cup water. Juices that contain pulp have a lower glycemic response, for example, Tropicana Grovestand Orange has a very high pulp content.)

TYPES OF DRINKS:

Liquid Boxed
Motts—Mini Orange Juice
Minute Maid 100% Orange Juice

Sports
Ener-G, Electrolyte Replace
Sports drinks made without:
    Maltodextrins
    Glucose polymers
    Corn syrup
    Sugar (sucrose)
    High fructose corn syrup

Soda/Soft Drinks
Sodas and diet drinks made without:
    Maltodextrins
    Glucose polymers
    Corn syrup
    Sugar (sucrose)
    High fructose corn syrup
Club soda
Seltzer
Tonic water (sugar-free)
Flavored waters without:
    high-glycemic sugars

Coffee/Tea
Coffee, ground or instant
    black without high-glycemic sugars
Tea, from tea bags
Loose tea

Coffee Creamers
Nature's First Natural Dairy Creamer

Hot Cocoa Mixes
Swiss Miss Fat Free
Carnation Fat Free
Carnation No Sugar Added

Vegetables
(Fresh or frozen)
Artichoke
Arugula
Asparagus
Avocado
Broccoli
Brussels sprouts
Cabbage, any type
Cauliflower
Celery
Collard greens
Eggplant
Endive
Escarole
Garlic
Green pepper
Red bell pepper
Yellow bell pepper
Kale
Kohlrabi
Leeks
Lettuce
Mushrooms
Mustard greens
Okra
Olives
Onions
Peppers, hot
Pickles
Radishes
Sauerkraut
Scallions

Spinach

Squash, summer yellow

Sweet potatoes or yams

Tomatoes

Turnip greens

Water chestnuts

Zucchini

Beans and Peas

Baked beans, canned

Black beans, fresh or frozen

Beans, green, wax, or Italian

Bean sprouts

Black-eyed peas, fresh or frozen

Butterbeans, fresh, frozen, or canned

Chickpeas, fresh or canned (higher)

Garbanzo, fresh or canned

Kidney beans, fresh or canned

Lentils (Dal Bengal gram) or red lentil

Lima beans, small

Pinto beans

Navy beans

Peas—yellow, green, split, dried, or
   frozen (dried are lowest)

Pea pods

Peanuts

Snow peas

Soybeans, dried or canned

White haricot, dried

Salads

Avocado salad

Caesar salad

Chef's salad

Cobb salad

Cole slaw (no carrots)

Egg salad (with hard-boiled egg,
   mayonnaise, celery, pickles, or dill relish)

Fruit salad (acceptable fruits only)

Green salad (no carrots)

Pasta salad (fresh)

Spinach salad

Shrimp or seafood salad

Tuna salad (with onions, celery, apple,
   pickles, or dill relish, lemon juice,
   and mayonnaise)

Vegetable salad (acceptable vegetables only)

Salsa

Newman's Own All Natural Salsa

Taco Bell Home Originals
   Thick 'n Chunky Salsa

Tostitos All Natural Salsa

Grains

Buckwheat kasha

Bulgar

Barley

Rye

Wheat kernels

Bottled Salad Dressing (2 Tbs.)
**(Don't assume that dressings labeled "Lite"
or "Fat-free" are automatically acceptable.
Some add corn syrup, maltodextrins, and
other high-glycemic ingredients.)**

Brianna's Homestyle
   Real French Vinaigrette

Cardini's Zesty Garlic

Hellmann's Creamy Caesar

Hellmann's Creamy Ranch

Ken's Chunky Blue Cheese

Ken's Ranch

Kraft Garlic Ranch

Kraft Balsamic Vinaigrette

Kraft Creamy Roasted Garlic

Newman's Own Caesar

Seven Seas Free Viva Italian

Wishbone Lite Italian

Wishbone Fat-free Italian

Spices/ Seasonings

Herbs such as basil, oregano, thyme,
    parsley, cilantro, dill, and bay leaf

Soy sauce

Spices such as black pepper, cayenne,
    pepper, cinnamon, nutmeg, and
    coriander

Low salt beef and chicken broth

Catsup (2–3 tsp. with protein)

Mustard

Salsa—see list

Hoagie spread

Fats, Oils, Butter, Mayonnaise

**(Most fats, oils, butters, and mayonnaise
are glycemically acceptable—but that does
not mean they are healthy choices. The following are the best choices.)**

Canola oil

Corn oil

Olive oil

Hellmann's Light Mayonnaise

I Can't Believe It's Not Butter!
    (spray, not solid)

Kraft Light Mayonnaise

Smart Balance Soft Spread
    (no trans-fatty acids)

Unsaturated corn oil

Margarine

Breads, Cookies, Cakes, Crackers

Ak-Mak 100% Stone Ground Whole
    Wheat Cracker

Alvarado Farms 100% Sprouted
    Wheat Bread

Alvarado Farms 100% Sprouted
    Wheat Bagel

Barley, coarse

Braunschlaggar European Style
    Rye Bread

Bulgar bread

Shiloh Farms 100% Whole Grain
    Wheat Bread

Shiloh Farms 100% Whole Grain
    Sprouted Wheat Bread

Shiloh Farms 100% Whole Grain
    Cracked Wheat Bread

Multi-grain, 9-grain

Nature's Choice Real Fruit Bar

Nature's Warehouse Juice-flavored
    Pastry Popover

Oat Bran Bread

Pita Bread (Alvarado Farms Sprouted
    Wheat), regular pita bread is borderline

Pound Cake (small slice)

Pumpernickel (Rye pumpernickel is
    lowest)

Rye bread (rye flour should be first
    ingredient)

Rye, coarse European style or whole
    grain or rye kernel or 100% whole
    grain rye bread

R. W. Frookie Fructose Cookie

Soda crackers

Sponge cake

Tortillas (wheat, not corn)

Cereal

All Bran, Regular and Fruit 'n Oats

Rice Bran

Bran Buds

Buckwheat, cooked

Buckwheat Kashi

Fiberwise

General Mills Fiber One

Healthy Start Cereal

Old-fashioned Quaker Oats Oatmeal
   (6 minutes cooking time)

Pearled Barley Cereal

Special K

Pastas

(Pastas vary in glycemic response, but most are in the acceptable range. Spaghetti and long pastas are lower than macaroni or small shaped pastas. The glycemic response goes up when over-boiled, so serve al dente. Use high-protein pasta (10+ grams of protein per serving) when possible.)

Brown rice pasta

Capellini

Fettuccine

Linguini

Lo mein, China Boy

Macaroni

Ravioli, cheese or meat filled

Rice Pasta

Spaghetti

Star

Tortellini, meat or cheese filled

Vermicelli (not rice vermicelli)

Brand Name Pastas

Contadina Spinach Linguini

Contadina Lemon Dill Angel Hair

Nutri-Mac Spaghetti

Pasta Sauces

(Sauces made without corn syrup, sugar, or any ingredient listed on the Unacceptable Foods List.)

Rice

(The glycemic index of rice varies from type to type. It is best to eat longer-grained rice, and basmati rice is your best choice. Like pasta, rice will have a lower glycemic index if it is not overcooked.)

Long grain—low glycemic
   Basmati—best choice
   Doongara—2nd best choice

Dairy

Buttermilk

Milk: whole, skim, low-fat, 2%

Cheese (Alpine Lace, Free 'n Lean
   Lite-Line)

Chocolate milk, low-fat

Cottage cheese, reg. and low-fat

Cream cheese, Philadelphia Lite Whipped

Custard, vanilla made with milk

Parmesan cheese, grated
   (not diet parmesan)

Sour cream, regular, low-fat, and nonfat

Soy milk, without sugars

Yogurt, low-fat or nonfat
   sugar-free without maltodextrins

Yogurt, Dannon Lite Fruit

Ice Cream, Frozen Dessert

(Ingredients vary. Look for low-fat brands without maltodextrins, glycose polymers, corn syrups, and dextrins.)

Creamsicles, low-fat or nonfat
   artificially sweetened
Frozen Yogurt, Baskin-Robbins
   sugar-free, nonfat
Frozen Yogurt, nonfat without maltodextrins
   and/or corn syrup
Ice cream, low-fat
Popsicles, sugar-free
Tropicana Fruit Juice Bars, fat-free
   no sugar added
I Can't Believe It's Yogurt—Yoglace

Snacks

Fig Newtons (2)
Health Valley Apple Muffins (1)
Gelatins and puddings (not instant) without
   maltodextrins or high-glycemic sugars
Nuts
Sugar-free gum

Soups

Campbell's Healthy Request:
   Chicken Noodle
   Minestrone
   Tomato
Nile Spice:
   Couscous Vegetable
   Chicken Soup with Almonds
   Couscous Lentil Curry
Progresso:
   Vegetable
Manhattan clam chowder
Chili
Shrimp or seafood gumbo

Jambalaya
Onion soup
Lentil soup
Gazpacho
Bouillabaisse
Fish soups (without potato)
Italian minestrone
Tomato soup
Bean and pasta soup, fresh only

Nutrition and Sports Bars

Pure Protein Bar/Worldwide Sports
 Nutrition

Diabetic Bars

The "G" Bar/Low-glycemic bar for
   diabetics

Chinese Food

(Chinese food has the lowest glycemic response of all takeout or restaurant food— do not eat the rice.)

Crab meat soup
Asparagus soup
Hot and sour soup
Watercress soup
Moo goo gai pan
Chinese bean thread
Chinese noodles (not fried)
Chicken with broccoli
Chicken or shrimp with Chinese veggies
   (no carrots or baby corn)
Lo mein
BBQ pork appetizer
Stir-fried green beans
Chicken in foil
Fish and seafood dishes (no carrots or
   baby corn)

Proteins

(Most proteins, such as seafood, poultry, turkey, beef, and tofu, are low glycemic. The exception is protein packaged or cooked with high-glycemic ingredients, such as meat dipped in flour and fried. The following categories are a list of acceptable protein from plants and animals.)

Plant Proteins

Soybeans

Whole soy products with fiber intact

Legumes

Nuts

Whole grains

Low-glycemic Meat Alternatives

Gardenburger Soy Burger

Green Giant Harvest
    Burgers for Recipes, all-vegetable
    protein crumbles

Veja-Links, Worthington vegetarian
    hotdogs

Meat, Poultry, and Fish
Best Nonplant Protein

Egg

Dairy products (low-fat)

Fish and shellfish

Poultry and game (skinless)

Pork (lean)

Beef (lean)

Goat

Mutton

GLYCEMICALLY UNACCEPTABLE FOODS

Fruit

Applesauce with sugar or corn syrup

Apricots, fresh or canned

Banana, yellow and ripe

Dates

Fruit cocktail (any)

Kiwi, very ripe

Mango

Paw paw

Papaya, ripe

Pineapple

Prunes

Pumpkin

Raisins

Sultanas

Watermelon

Canned Fruit

Fruit in light or heavy syrup

Del Monte:

    Lite Peach Cup

    Lite Pear Cup

    Fruit Cup

    Lite Fruit Cocktail

    Chunky Mixed Fruit in heavy syrup

    Lite Pear Halves in extra-lite syrup

    Peach Halves in heavy syrup

Mott's:

    Fruitsations

    Homestyle Chunky Applesauce with

      brown sugar

White House:

    Applesauce

    Cinnamon Applesauce

Juices
(Fresh, canned, bottled, or frozen.)

Beet juice

Carrot juice

Celery juice

Prune juice

Watermelon juice

White and red grape juice

Juices made from high-glycemic fruits

    and juices sweetened with high-

    glycemic sugars

Juice and Drink Mixes

Country Time Sugar-Free Pink:

    Lemonade

Crystal Light:

    Raspberry Tea

    Pink Lemonade

    Lemonade

    Pineapple Orange Banana

    Peach

    Body Refreshers (regular)

Kool-Aid:

    Sugar-free

    Regular Nonsweetened

Box Drinks
(These drinks are not acceptable because they are sweetened either with sugar or with aspertame.)

Arizona Ice Tea (regular)

Arizona Green Tea

Capri Sun All-Natural:

    Mountain Cooler

    Orange

Wild Cherry

Strawberry Kiwi

Grape

Hawaiian Punch

Hershey Chocolate Drink

Hi-C

Minute Maid All Natural Berry Punch

Soda, Soft Drinks

Colas, sodas and drinks made with any

high-glycemic sugars or carbohydrates

Auntie Anne's (in the mall):

Dutch Ice

Kiwi Banana

Orange Creme

Lemonade

Raspberry

Mocha

Strawberry

Fanta

Coffee

Instant coffees made with high-glycemic

ingredients

Tea

Bagged or loose hot tea

Lipton Natural Brew:

Iced Tea Mix

Diet Peach

Diet Lemon

Diet Raspberry

Nestea:

Lemon Bliss Herb Tea

Instant

Decaf

Sugar-Free

Coffee Creamers

Borden Cremora:

Royale Nondairy Creamer

Rich 'n Creamy Lite Nondairy

Creamer

Fat-free Nondairy Creamer

Nestle Carnation:

Coffee Mate (regular)

French Vanilla Coffee Mate

Hazelnut Coffee Mate

Fat-free Nondairy Creamer

Hot Cocoa Mixes (dry-powdered)

Carnation:

Milk Chocolate with Mini

Marshmallows

Rich Chocolate

Malted Milk

Nestle's Quick:

Chocolate

Chocolate with No Sugar Added

Ovaltine:

Rich Chocolate

Chocolate Malt

Malt

Swiss Miss:

Lite

Marshmallow Lovers

Chocolate Sensation

Milk Chocolate

Bottled Drinks

Hawaiian Punch Fruit Juicy Red

Kool-Aid Bursts:

Blastin Berry Cherry

Tropical Punch

Slammin Strawberry Kiwi

Great Blue Dini

Libby's:

    Peach, Pear, or Apricot Nectar

Pedialyte, unflavored

Squeezit Berry B. Wild

Tropicana Twister:

    Grape Berry

    Strawberry Kiwi

    Tropical Fruit

Troppi Tropical Punch

Twister, regular

V8 Splash Strawberry Kiwi

V8 Splash Berry Blend

Water (flavored waters) with sugar or

    high-glycemic ingredients

Sports Drinks (powder mixes)

Gatorade:

    Orange

    Lemon Lime

Sports Drinks (bottled)

Gatorade:

    Cherry Rush

    Cool Blue Raspberry

    Fruit Punch

    Strawberry Kiwi

    Lemon Ice

    Citrus Cooler

    Frost

Powerade, regular

Sportsplus

All drinks with maltodextrins or glucose

    polymers

Vegetables

Beets

Carrots

Corn—canned, fresh, frozen

Parsnips

Pillsbury Idaho Mashed

    Potatoes (granules)

Potatoes—canned, new, baked, mashed,

    instant, French fries, chips. Baked,

    mashed, sliced, microwaved, or boiled.

    (The lowest glycemic and low-fat way

    to fix potatoes is to boil them, drain,

    cut open, and spray with olive oil or I

    Can't Believe It's Not Butter! Don't

    eat potatoes alone. Eat them with

    proteins, i.e., chicken, fish, or meat

    and a vegetable.)

Beans

Broad beans

Fava beans

Nutrition Bars, Diabetic Bars, Sports Bars

Meade Johnson Nutritional's Choice

    Bar

Kudos whole grain bars

Muesli bars, fruit

Power Bar

Zone Force Bar, 40%-30%-30%

Breads

Bagel, regular

Biscuits

Bread, gluten-free

Bread stuffing

Breadsticks, Italian and regular

Buns—hamburger and hot dog

Corn bread

Croissant

Croutons

English muffin

French baguette (plain or wheat)

Kaiser rolls

Muffins—berry or bran

Pancakes

Pumpernickel

Rye, commercial American

Rye, dark or light

White bread or rolls

White wheat or whole wheat bread

Whole meal bread

Sourdough bread

Cookies, Cakes, Crackers

Angel food cake

Crispbread

Donuts

Melba toast

Rice cakes

Rye, crisp bread or whole meal

Ryvita crackers

Richard Simmons:

   Lowfat Strawberry Marshmallow

     Sandwich Cookies

   97% Fat-free Chocolate

     Devil's Food Cookies

Stoned Wheat Thins

Taco shells

Vanilla Wafers

Waffles

Wheat crackers

Cereals (cold)

Bran Chex

40% Bran Flakes

Cheerios

Coco Pops

Corn Bran

Corn Chex

Cornflakes

Crispix

Grape-Nuts

Honey Smacks

Life

Mini-Wheats

Muesli, non-toasted

Nutri Grain

100% Oat Bran

Post Flakes

Puffed Kashi

Puffed Rice or Wheat

Rice Chex

Rice Crispies

Shredded Wheat

Sultana Bran

Sustain

Team

Total

Wheetabix

Cereals (hot)

Cream of Wheat or Rice

Muesli or Muesli Bars

Oat Bran Flakes

Oatmeal, instant

Oatmeal Porridge

Porridge Oats

Ready-to-eat processed cereals

Rolled Oats

Tapioca, cooked

Wheatens

Wheat or Rice, precooked

Pasta Sauces

(Canned or homemade with sugar, honey, corn syrup, maltodextrins, or high fructose corn syrup.)

Pasta

Canned pasta

Canned noodles

Gnocchi

Macaroni and cheese
    canned or packaged

Rice pasta

Rice vermicelli

Spaghetti O's

Pasta cooked for too long

Rice

(Avoid short-grain rice in general, since they have a higher glycemic index.)

Asian rice

Brown rice

Glutenous rice

Instant rice

White rice

Rice A Roni

Rice cakes

Rice drinks

Sticky rice

Tapioca

Waxy rice

Wild rice

Grains

Couscous

Millet

Dairy

Cool Whip:
    regular
    lite

Instant pudding mixes

Parmesan cheese "free" nonfat grated topping

Sweetened condensed whole milk

Ice Cream, Frozen Desserts

(Many fat-free frozen desserts are not acceptable. They raise blood sugar more than high-fat desserts.)

High-fat ice cream

Bryers No Sugar Added
    Light Ice Cream

D'Lites Ice Cream, Fat-free

Haagen-Dazs:
    Zesty Lemon Sorbet
    Chocolate Sorbet

TCBY, No Sugar Added Nonfat

TCBY, Frozen Sorbet

Tofu ice cream or frozen dessert

Ice Cream Toppings

Hershey's Syrup, Chocolate Fat-free

Smucker's Toppings:
    Walnuts in Syrup
    Hot Fudge

Fats, Oils

Butter

Coconut oil

Palm Kernel oil

Palm oil

Saturated fats

Snacks

Candy bars

Corn chips

Jelly beans, regular, nondiet

Life Savers, regular

Popcorn—cakes, theater, packaged, air-
    popped, low-fat, fat-free, microwave,
    cheese-flavored

Potato chips, fried or baked

Pretzels

Rice cakes

THE THREE FOOD GROUPS

It is not only important to eat a low-glycemic diet, but also to eat mixed meals in proper proportions of carbohydrates, protein, and fat. I have found that the percentages that work best are 55 percent low-glycemic carbohydrates, 20 percent lean protein, and 25 percent acceptable fat.

CARBOHYDRATES

To some people, 55 percent carbohydrates might seem an intimidating amount. After reading some of the popular diet books on the market today, many people have shifted their dietary fears from fat to carbohydrates. The key is not fearing carbohydrates, but learning how to manage them in all forms relative to your activity level. You may have friends who are losing large amounts of scale weight on low carbohydrate diets, but I'm willing to bet a month's pay that they look drawn in the face and feel headachy and fatigued all the time. The reason for this is simple: To maintain the brain and central nervous system, the body needs a certain amount of glucose, which it gets from sugars and starches, the by-products of carbohydrates after digestion. The body stores this glucose in the liver and in the muscles. If you are not eating enough carbs, the body has to get its supply from somewhere. What happens then is that the body begins breaking down muscle protein to synthesize glucose to supply your vital organs with an adequate supply. You will lose weight, but it will be muscle, not fat, because your body cannot break down its fat stores into glycogen.

The goal of a good weight loss program should always be to lose as little muscle as possible in comparison to fat loss. For every gram of muscle tissue, you lose 4 grams of water. For every gram of fat lost, you lose only 1 gram of water. Losing water weight does not represent true long-term weight loss because water is the easiest thing in the world to gain back. When you begin increasing your carbohydrate intake during times of stress eating, the body regains lost muscle tissue and its associated water weight. Of course, we are talking about losing water weight over the long term. Everyone is somewhat dehydrated after vigorous exercise, but that water is easily replaced by simply drinking fluids.

Also, exercising while on a low carbohydrate diet increases the metabolic process of muscle breakdown. The solution is not to stop exercising, but to take advantage of the positive fat-burning effects of exercise and adjust your calories (and therefore your energy from carbohydrates) up or down, relative to your activity level. Exercise is always factored into the amount of calories you ingest.

Remember, the goal of any diet and exercise program should be to spare lean muscle tissue at the expense of excess body fat. So, don't fear carbohydrates. Eaten in the proper amounts, they can be your new best friend. That does not mean, however, that you can eat all the carbohydrates you want, just as you couldn't eat all the fat you want or all the sugar you want without paying the consequences. A recent study at Stanford University School of Medicine showed that eating a diet extremely high in carbohydrates caused triglycerides (bad fats) to go up. It is possible to have too much of a good thing. The key is balance.

PROTEIN

I suggest making lean protein sources 20 percent of your food intake. From a dietary standpoint, protein is a stabilizing tool that assists in insulin management, as well as serving other vital roles in normal body function. But protein is not stored. Therefore, to keep insulin in check, a person requires three balanced meals and two or three snacks that include protein per day to suppress hunger and mobilize body fat for burning during physical activity. A good protein snack food would be fat metabolizer soy-based foods such as Personal Edge® soy powder, which you can find in many health food stores or General Nutrition Stores in your area, by calling (877) 982-3343, or by visiting the Web site www.personaledgeprotein.com. I suggest ½ serving in low-fat milk or unsweetened, glycemically acceptable orange juice, twice daily.

Soy foods have always been a part of my fitness and nutrition programs because of their many benefits to the human body. Scientific studies have shown that an overabundance of the amino acid lysine increases bad cholesterol, while the amino acid arginine decreases it. Compared to casein (animal protein), soy has a more favorable arginine to lysine ratio. This lower ratio also decreases the body's production of insulin and increases its production of glucagon. In other words, having soy every day helps you to shift your fat metabolism from insulin storage to insulin mobilization.

Soy protein also helps to lower the risk of coronary disease and is an important part of a total fat and cholesterol-lowering program when used in conjunction with a properly balanced nutrition and aerobic exercise program. Soy foods have also been known to lower the risk for hormone-related cancers.

Besides soy-based powders, there are many delicious soy food products available, including soy burgers, hot dogs, soy milk, and soy cheese. Vegetarians can take advantage of soy foods to make sure that they get enough protein in their diet.

When choosing other protein sources, always choose lean meats and low-fat dairy. First-choice protein sources include skim milk; fat-free cheese and cottage cheese; yogurt made from skim milk; 95 percent lean ground beef, turkey, or encased meats (sausage, bologna, etc.); white meat, skinless chicken; white-meat tuna in water; egg whites; and nonfried fish and seafood.

The *American Journal of Clinical Nutrition* states that eating fish daily decreases insulin, increases glucose production, lowers triglyceride (bad fat) production, and increases the level of HDL2 cholesterol (good cholesterol), reducing the risk of cardiovascular disease. While I don't insist that you eat freshwater fish daily, it is important to eat it at least twice a week.

While the current RDA recommendation for protein is 0.8 grams per kilograms of body weight, this does not provide enough for the needs of individuals who engage in regular exercise. I agree with well-known diet author Barry Sears, Ph. D., that basing protein needs on total body weight is an inaccurate measurement. Body weight is made of fat-free weight (lean body mass, bone, and blood) and fat weight (metabolically inactive tissue). Why should we feed metabolically inactive tissue?

Many books give you complicated mathematical formulas to figure out how much protein you need per day. I have done the work for you in the meal plans that come later in this chapter. (See pgs. pages 72–78.)

Getting adequate protein in your diet is important for another reason. A recent article in *The Journal of Clinical Endocrinology and Metabolism* reports that "Diets low in protein lead to increases in sex hormone-binding globulin in older men, potentially reducing the availability of testosterone and causing loss of muscle mass, red cell mass and bone density." Based on a study of men between the ages of 40 and 70 years, this article suggests that eating a diet with adequate amounts of protein helps stop the decrease in testosterone levels that many men experience as they age.

FATS

Most people think that all fat is bad, but this is not so. By having 25 percent of our diet as the right kind of fat, we can use dietary fat to help burn body fat. All fats produce 9 calories of energy per gram. The body uses fats mostly as an energy source, along with the glucose broken down from the digestion of carbohydrates. There are two different groups of fat. The first is saturated, which is usually found in meat and dairy products such as beef, cheese, and butter. It is important to eat saturated fats in limited amounts because a diet containing too many saturated fats will clog up your arteries and increase your chances of heart disease. Eating foods high in saturated fats has also been linked to a greater risk of cancer.

The second type of fat is unsaturated, which comes from plant products and includes foods such as vegetable oils, nuts, and avocados. Your body uses this type of fat primarily to strengthen cell membranes, to support nerve and hormone function, and to produce hormonelike substances called prostaglandins, which have been linked to the prevention of heart disease and cancers.

One category of unsaturated fat that your body needs to survive are the essential fatty acids omega-6 (linoleic acid) and omega-3 (alpha linolenic acid). Your body cannot make these fatty acids, so you must obtain them from your diet. Omega-6 is fairly common and is found in most of the vegetable oils sold in the grocery store. The problem with typical grocery store oils, however, is that they are processed for mass distribution, which means that they are often filled with free radicals and a bad fat called trans-fatty acid. Omega-3 can be fund in canola, flaxseed soy, and walnut oils, and in dark green, leafy vegetables.

Although the ideal ratio of omega-6 oil to omega-3 is between 3:1 and 4:1, most people in this country have twenty times the level of omega-6 than omega-3 because the American diet is so deficient in the latter. Therefore, I recommend supplementing your diet with omega-3 oils. Benefits of this (and the subsequent increase in protaglandins in the body) include:

- Lowering of cholesterol levels
- Prevention of strokes and heart attacks
- Decrease of symptoms of angina
- Lowering of high blood pressure
- Improvement of rheumatoid arthritis
- Decrease of symptoms of multiple sclerosis
- Improvement in the skin conditions psoriasis and eczema
- Prevention and treatment of cancer

Besides the ones I have mentioned above, there are several other ways that you can increase the amount of essential fatty acids in your diet. Cold-water fish such as salmon, trout, and mackeral are rich sources of the essential fatty acid metabolites DHA (docosahexaenoic acid) and EPA (eicosapen-taenoic acid), which have been implicated in lowering blood pressure and improving cholesterol levels. A good way to supplement your diet with omega-3 is by taking fish oil capsules, which are available at most pharmacies or health food stores.

Flax oil is, by far, the richest source of omega-3 and all essential fatty acids, which is why body builders mix it into their protein drinks so often. It is also much less expensive than other supplements containing fatty acids. A month's supple of fish oils costs $70, and a month's supply of evening primrose oil costs $90, while flaxseed oil will only cost you $12 per month. Flaxseed oil has the added advantage of being converted by bacteria in the gut into lignans, special compounds that have impressive health benefits. These benefits include anticancer, antibacterial, antifungal, and antiviral abilities.

It is best not to take flaxseed oil in capsules, but in liquid form to make sure that it is fresh and of high quality. Flaxseed oil is very delicate and can go bad if not processed or stored correctly. Not all oils are prepared the same way, or at the same temperatures, and taste is the only way you can tell if you have a good product. High quality flaxseed oil will have a delicious, nutty flavor, while oils that have been damaged or gone rancid will have a bitter taste due to the presence of lipid peroxides—toxic molecules that can do bodily harm.

The next time you are fixing a green salad, try using a tablespoon of flax oil as a dressing, or half a tablespoon mixed with sunflower oil or a little vinegar. If you are eating out at a restaurant that doesn't have flaxseed oil, ask for some olive oil, canola oil, or sunflower oil for your salad. It's usually not a good idea to cook with flaxseed oil since it is heat and light sensitive, but it is very tasty when lightly brushed over meat after it has been cooked. A bit of walnut oil or flax oil gives a nice taste to a dry chicken breast. You might also add walnuts, almonds, or sunflower seeds to your nutrition plan, but do so in moderation since these nuts are high in calories.

When increasing your essential fatty acid intake, you should also take 400 I.U. (international units) of vitamin E, 500 mg of vitamin C, and 200 mcg of selenium to provide balance in your body. When fats are broken down in our bodies, they can release free radicals, also known as "oxidents," which have been known to damage cell structure and can lead to premature aging and increase your chances of developing diseases such as cancer. These vitamins, which are all present in the proper amounts in any good anti-oxident supplement, will help your body to neutralize these free radicals. Consider consulting with a registered dietitian to provide you with the appropriate vitamin E and essential fatty acid ratios relative to your individual nutritional requirements.

Other acceptable oils include corn oil, Hellman's Light Mayonnaise, Kraft Light Mayonnaise, Smart Balance Soft Spread (no trans fats), and unsaturated corn oil. Promise, Take Control, Fleischmann's Margarine, and I Can't Believe It's Not Butter! (spray, not solid) are excellent butter alternatives. When dining out, if real butter is your only choice, use it in moderation.

THE VALUE OF FIBER

Fiber is any plant food that passes undigested through the small intestine. There are two basic types of fiber, insoluble and soluble. Insoluble fibers hold less water than the soluble ones and include foods such as whole grains, vegetables, and most brans. They provide the bulk of stool and help to normalize bowel movements. Soluble fibers hold up to forty times their weight in water and include such foods as psyllium, legumes, and oats. This type of fiber provides the primary food source for friendly bacteria in the intestinal track. When we do not get enough soluble fiber, this can lead to constipation, reduced growth of friendly bacteria, increased growth of unfriendly bacteria, and an increased risk of colorectal cancer. Apples and citrus (pectins) are the most soluble fibers, holding one hundred times their weight in water.

According to a recent article in the *Journal of the American Medical Association,* eating a high-fiber diet helps us to fight obesity. Young adults who ate at least 21 grams of fiber per day gained, on an average, 8 pounds less over a 10-year period than those who ate the least amount of fiber. Getting sufficient fiber is not that hard when you realize that a bowl of high-fiber cereal can contain up to 25 grams.

Another great benefit we get from eating sufficient fiber is that it slows down the rate of nutrient absorption following a meal, reducing our blood sugar levels and our body's secretion of insulin. So, if you want to stabilize your body's insulin response, fiber is one of your allies.

Although the average American eats between 16 and 17 grams of fiber per day, the National Cancer Institute recommends eating an average of 25 grams daily. However, a recent study by the American Diabetes Association has led the American Dietary Association to begin work revising its dietary recommendations of fiber *upward*. In this study, diabetics were shown to significantly reduce their blood sugar—and even get off their medication—by eating up to 50 grams of fiber per day. Other benefits of this high-fiber diet were an improved cholesterol level, which lowered the participants' risk of heart disease, a major cause of death among diabetics (and the number one cause of death in the overall American population).

Eating a diet high in fiber also helps prevent peptic ulcers, irritable bowel syndrome, hiatal hernias, inflamatory bowel diseases, gallbladder disease, and hemorrhoids.

Types of high-fiber foods include:

- Whole grains, such as whole wheat, whole or rolled oats, buckwheat, amaranth, and brown rice.
- Breads, cereals, and rolls made from whole grain flour.
- Raw fruits such as apples (skins on) and dried fruits such as apricots, figs, prunes, raisins, and dates. (Try to buy organic dried fruits because the drying process tends to concentrate the level of fungicides and pesticides.)
- Raw or slightly cooked vegetables.
- All nuts, beans, peas, lentils, potatoes, and yams (with their skins on).

When you increase the amount of fiber that you eat daily, make sure that you do this slowly to avoid discomfort and flatulence. Also make sure to take a multivitamin since fiber speeds digestion and can deplete the body of some vitamins.

A WORD ABOUT LOW-FAT FOODS, SUGAR, AND SUGAR SUBSTITUTES[4]

As many of us strive to lose weight, we often fill our shopping carts with "fat-free" foods. This may sound like a good plan, but Dr. Ann de Wees Allen of the Glycemic Institute warns that such labeling is highly deceiving:

As sugars and carbohydrates filled the empty space that fats left in packaged food, their fat-storing properties increase dramatically. Manufacturers rushed to remove the fats from their prepared food and reengineered them into fat-free, more "healthy" foods. The irony is that the fats in the foods are not as fattening as the sugars which have replaced them. As a result, many of the "fat-free" foods are actually much more fattening than they were before the fat was removed.

It is also true that all sugars are not created equal. "Bad" sugars include maltodextrins, glucose and glucose polymers, invert sugar, dextrose, raw sugars, honey, brown sugar, barley malt, date sugar, turbinado sugar, cane sugar, maple sugar, carmelized sugar, and blackstrap molasses. All of these sugars are high-glycemic and elevate blood sugar, making us more insulin resistant. While sucrose has a lower glycemic index than these other sugars, studies have shown that it has long-term negative health effects and has actually been shown to increase the risk of heart disease in 20 percent of the population due to elevated serum triglyceride levels.

So, read the ingredients on the processed foods and low-fat desserts before you buy these products. You may be disappointed to realize that you are filling your kitchen with "diet" foods that cause you to actually *gain* weight, not *lose* it. Research has shown that high-glycemic sugars also work to suppress the immune system. As Dr. Allen puts it, cancer cells thrive on these kinds of sugars.

Fortunately, there are natural, low-glycemic sugars that do not stimulate fat storage or elevate blood sugar. Foods sweetened with fruit sugars made from low-glycemic fruits are your best choice. If you want to know if a food product has been sweetened with fruit sugars—and what kind of fruit—simply read the label. It will be listed as one of the ingredients.

Finally, it is important to realize that not all artificial sweeteners are created equal. Some are mixed with high-glycemic ingredients when they are packaged. For example, Equal is mixed with dextrose and maltodextrins, which are high-glycemic fillers. Maybe one tiny serving of these kinds of sweeteners might not have a negative impact on your blood sugar, but several servings during the course of the day surely will. Low-glycemic artificial sweetners include NutraSweet, saccharin, cyclamate, Sunette, Sweet-One, Maltitol, and Sucralose. Artificial sweeteners that include high-glycemic fillers include Sweet Thing and Sweet 'N Low.

COMPUTING HOW MANY CALORIES
YOU WILL NEED PER DAY

Now that you know *what kinds* of foods to eat, the questions becomes *how much?* Although men should never go below 1,650 calories per day, to keep your body from going into fat-storage famine mode, you will have days when your caloric needs are higher relative to the amount of physical activity you are engaging in. To lose weight, you should eat about 500 calories less per day than what you actually need to match your activity level. A chart that lists the amount of calories expended in certain sports and activities can be found on page 61.

Estimating your daily caloric requirements is fairly easy. I am going to offer you a choice of two methods for determining which category you fit into: (1) the 2,000 calorie-per-day diet, (2) the 1,800-calorie-per-day diet, or (3) the 1,650-calorie-per-day diet. The first method requires a bit more math. The second, developed by Molly Kimball, a licensed, registered nutritionist, is clean, simple, and equally effective.

CRITERIA FOR DETERMINING CALORIC NEEDS, METHOD #1

Step 1: Determine your resting metabolic rate (RMR) by multiplying your body weight by 10. If you are a 140-pound man, you would start with 1,400 calories.

$$140 \times 10 = 1,400$$

Step 2: Calculate how many calories you will need for purposeful exercise. If you plan on walking for 30 minutes, you would calculate how many calories you would expend by multiplying the amount of calories/hour/pound of body fat expended by this exercise (see Figure 3.1 on page 61) and multiplying that by your weight. Then divide by 2 because it's only half an hour.

$$\frac{2.4 \text{ calories/hour (expended walking)} \times 140 \text{ pounds}}{2}$$

Add the answer, 168 calories, to 1,400 to get 1,568 calories.

You can add in an hour-long game of volleyball using the same formula, except for dividing by 2 because this is an hour-long activity.

2.2 calories/hour (expended playing volleyball) X 140 pounds

That will give you an additional 308 calories. Add this number to 1,568 to get 1,876 calories.

Step 3: Determine how many calories you will need for your day's activities in addition to your purposeful exercise. If you are going to be mostly sedentary, add in 20 percent to 40 percent of your RMR. If you plan on being moderately active, then add in 40 percent to 60 percent of your RMR. If you will be very active, add in 60 percent to 80 percent of your RMR.

Walking for half an hour and playing volleyball for an hour might be thought of as moderately active, so you would add in 560 calories.

1,400 (RMR) X 40% = 560 calories

Adding them all up, you would need 560 calories + 1,876 calories = 2,436 calories to remain at the exact same weight. Theoretically, if you eat 500 calories a day less than what you need, you will lose about a pound a week. If you eat a glycemically correct meal, your body will go into your fat stores to retrieve most of the extra energy you will need, and you will probably lose even more.

Below is a chart that gives you the calories you will burn engaging in specific activities.

Activity	Calories/hour/pound body weight
Aerobics, high impact	3.2
Aerobics, low impact	2.3
Badminton	2.6
Basketball, game	3.6
Basketball, shooting baskets	2.0
Bicycling, 10 mph	2.7
Bicycling, stationary, moderate effort	3.2
Bowling	1.4
Circuit training, general	3.6
Construction, outside remodeling	2.5

Activity	Calories/hour/pound body weight
Dancing, general	2.0
Fishing, general	1.8
Gardening, hoeing and digging	3.2
Golf, walking	2.3
Handball, general	5.4
Handball, team game	3.6
Hiking, hilly	3.6
Horseback riding	1.8
Jogging, 6 mph	4.2
Jumping rope	3.8
Kayaking	2.3
Painting, outside	2.1
Racewalking	2.9
Racquetball	4.1
Rope jumping, medium effort	4.6
Rowing machine	3.1
Scuba diving	3.8
Skating, ice	2.6
Skiing, cross-country	3.7
Skiing, downhill	2.6
Squash	4.3
Soccer	3.7
Stair, treadmill, general	2.7
Surfing	1.4
Swimming, fast/vigorous	4.5
Swimming, light/moderate	3.6
Table tennis	1.9
Tennis, singles	2.9
Tennis, doubles	1.8
Volleyball	2.2
Walking, 3.5 mph	2.4
Water skiing	3.0
Weight training	1.9

FIGURE 3.1: CALORIES BURNED DURING EXERCISE

CRITERIA FOR DETERMINING CALORIC NEEDS, METHOD #2

A simple and easy way to determine how many calories you need on an average day is to go by your frame size. You can use the following method to determine the size of your frame. Simply divide your height by your wrist circumference. Height is measured without shoes and wrist circumference is measured at the crease of the dominant wrist using a tape measure. In other words, if you are right handed, measure your right wrist.

Measuring Frame Size:

$$\frac{[\text{Height in centimeters (inches} \times 2.5)]}{\text{Wrist circumference in centimeters (inches} \times 2.5)}$$

[Here is an example of how this formula would work for a man who is 5' 10" tall (70 inches) and has a wrist circumference of 8 inches. Notice that you can convert inches to centimeters by multiplying them by 2.5]

Example of Measuring Frame Size:

$$\frac{[70 \text{ inches} \times 2.5 = 175 \text{ centimeters}]}{[8 \text{ inches} \times 2.5 = 20 \text{ centimeters}]}$$

= 8.75 centimeters

A measurement greater than 10.4 means that you have a small frame and should follow the 1,650 calorie per day meal plan. A measurement of 9.6 to 10.4 means you have a medium frame and should follow the 1,800 calorie per day meal plan. A measurement less than 9.6 means that you have a large frame and should follow the 2,000 calorie per day meal plan.

Once you have figured out how many calories per day you need to eat to lose weight, refer to the following chart to determine your servings per day of starch, fruit, milk, soy food products, vegetables, lean meats and fish, and fats, based upon 55 percent low-glycemic carbohydrates, 20 percent lean protein, and 25 percent acceptable fat.

MACKIE SHILSTONE
ABDOMINAL FAT LOSS PROGRAM
FOR MEN

Caloric Distribution:

55% Low-glycemic Carbohydrates; 20% Low-fat Protein; 25% Acceptable Fat

TOTAL SERVINGS PER DAY

	2,000 Calorie Diet	1,800 Calorie Diet	1,650 Calorie Diet
Starch	9	8	7
Fruit	5	5	4
Milk (skim)	2	2	2
Soy Food Product	1	1	1
Vegetables	4	4	3
Lean meat or fish	7	6	5
Fats	5	4	4

FIGURE 3.2: TOTAL SERVINGS PER DAY RELATIVE TO CALORIC INTAKE

DEVELOPING A DAILY MEAL PLAN USING PROPER PORTIONS

The numbers in the above chart refer to the *portions* of each type of food. Because foods vary in their caloric, carbohydrate, protein, and fat content, I have worked with nutritionist Molly Kimball to divide the foods that will make up your meal plan into six different groups. Each separate item listed is measured or weighed so that the amount of calories, carbohydrates, protein, and fat will be similar for all foods within a group. Added to this is a soy food product that can be included in your diet. Try to follow these portion guidelines when choosing foods from the Glycemically Acceptable List. This list contains many of your favorite brand names.

Starches and Breads: Each food listed contains about 15 grams of carbohydrate, 3 grams of protein, a trace of fat, and 80 calories.

Cereals—Grains—Pasta	1 serving
Bran cereal, dense (All Bran, Fiber One)	⅓ cup
Other cereals	¾ cup

Bulgar, cooked	½ cup
Oatmeal	½ cup
Pasta, cooked	½ cup
Rice, cooked	⅓ cup

Dried Beans—Peas—Lentils

Beans/ peas/ lentils, cooked	
(kidney, white, navy, split, black-eyed	⅓ cup
Baked beans	⅓ cup

Starchy Vegetables

Lima beans	½ cup
Green beans	½ cup
Yam, sweet potato	⅓ cup

Bread—Crackers

(100% whole wheat only)

Bagel	½ (1 oz.)
English muffin	½
Hot dog or hamburger bun	½
Pita, 6" across	½
Tortilla, 6" across	1
Plain roll, small	1 (1 oz.)
Bread, whole wheat	1 slice
Rye or pumpernickel	1 slice
Cracked wheat roll	1
Whole wheat crackers, fat free	4-6
Soda crackers	6

Meat and Meat Substitutes: Each serving of meat and meat substitutes contains approximately 7 grams of protein. The calories and amount of fat depend on the type of meat you choose. Two oz. of meat = 1 small chicken leg or thigh; 3 oz. of meat = 1 medium pork chop, 1 small hamburger, ½ of a whole chicken breast, or 1 fish fillet about the size of a deck of cards.

Lean Meat and Substitutes   1 serving

Beef

USDA select or choice grades

Lean beef—round, sirloin, flank steak,

    tenderloin, chipped beef   1 oz.

Pork

Lean pork—fresh ham, Canadian

    bacon, tenderloin   1 oz.

Veal

Veal chops and roasts (no cutlets)   1 oz.

Poultry

Skinless chicken, turkey, or Cornish hen   1 oz.

Fish

All fresh and frozen fish   1 oz.

Crab, lobster, shrimp, clams   2 oz.

Oysters   6 medium

Tuna, canned in water   1/4 cup

Cheese

Cottage cheese   1/4 cup

Grated parmesan   2 Tbsp.

Reduced-calorie cheese (<55 calories)   1 oz.

Other

Egg whites   3 whites

Egg substitutes (<55 calories per 1/2 cup)   1/2 cup

Medium-fat Meat and Substitutes   1 serving

Beef

Most beef products—all ground beef

    meatloaf, roasts (rib, chuck, rump),

    steak (cubed, T-bone)   1 oz.

Pork

Most pork pork products—chops, loin roast,
   cutlet   1 oz.

Veal

Cutlet (unbreaded)   1 oz.

Poultry

Chicken with skin, domestic duck
   or goose, ground turkey   1 oz.

Fish

Tuna (canned in oil and drained)   ¼ cup
Salmon (canned)   ¼ cup

Cheese—skim or part-skim

Ricotta   ¼ cup
Mozzarella   1 oz.
Reduced-calorie cheeses
   (56–80 calories per oz.)   1 oz.

Other

Lean luncheon meat   1 oz.
Egg   1
Egg substitutes (56–80 calories per ¼ cup)   ½ cup
Tofu   4 oz.

High-fat Meat and Substitutes   1 serving

(These are high in saturated fat, cholesterol, and calories and are strongly discouraged. Eat no more than once per week.)

Beef

Most USDA prime cuts of beef,
   ribs, corned beef   1 oz.

Pork

Spareribs, ground pork, pork sausage 1 oz.

Lamb

Patties—ground lamb 1 oz.

Cheese

All regular cheeses 1 oz.

Other

No-sugar peanut butter 1 Tbsp.

Vegetables: Each vegetable listed contains abut 5 grams of carbohydrate, 2 grams of protein, and 25 calories per serving. Vegetables contain 2 to 3 grams of fiber and are a great source of vitamins and minerals. One serving equals ½ cup cooked vegetable or juice or 1 cup of raw vegetables. If you are feeling hungry, however, these nonstarchy vegetables are so low in calories that you can have an extra serving to give yourself a feeling of fullness. Fresh and frozen vegetables should be your first choice. In some cases, frozen vegetables are even more nutrient-rich than fresh vegetables because they were frozen right after harvest and did not suffer a loss of nutrients during transit to the market. Canned vegetables are my last choice, but they are still acceptable. Just read the label on the can and make sure that it says "low sodium" or "no sodium." It is better to eat whole vegetables than juiced ones because juicing removes a significant amount of fiber.

Fresh—Frozen—Canned	1 serving
Artichoke (½ medium)	½ cup cooked, 1 cup raw
Asparagus	½ cup cooked, 1 cup raw
Beans (green, wax, Italian)	½ cup cooked, 1 cup raw
Bean sprouts	½ cup cooked, 1 cup raw
Broccoli	½ cup cooked, 1 cup raw
Brussel sprouts	½ cup cooked, 1 cup raw

Cabbage	½ cup cooked, 1 cup raw
Cauliflower	½ cup cooked, 1 cup raw
Eggplant	½ cup cooked, 1 cup raw
Greens (collard, mustard, turnip)	½ cup cooked, 1 cup raw
Mushrooms	½ cup cooked, 1 cup raw
Okra	½ cup cooked, 1 cup raw
Onions	½ cup cooked, 1 cup raw
Pea pods	½ cup cooked, 1 cup raw
Peppers (green)	½ cup cooked, 1 cup raw
Sauerkraut	½ cup cooked, 1 cup raw
Spinach	½ cup cooked, 1 cup raw
Summer squash	½ cup cooked, 1 cup raw
Tomato	½ cup cooked, 1 cup raw
Tomato/vegetable juice	1 cup
Water chestnuts	½ cup cooked, 1 cup raw
Zucchini	½ cup cooked, 1 cup raw

Fruits: Each fruit listed contains about 15 grams of carbohydrates and 60 calories. Most fruits have about 2 grams of fiber per serving. Whole fruit is a better choice than unsweetened canned juice because when fruits are juiced, they loose a significant amount of their fiber. If fruits are eaten dried, 1 serving equals ¼ cup.

Fresh—Frozen—Unsweetened Canned	**1 serving**
Apple (2 inches in diameter)	1
Applesauce (unsweetened)	½ cup
Banana (green)	½
Blackberries, blueberries	¾ cup
Cantaloupe, honeydew	1 cup
Figs (raw)	2
Grapefruit (medium)	½
Kiwi (large, not very ripe)	1
Mandarin oranges	1
Nectarine (2 ½ inches in diameter)	1
Peach (small)	1 or ¾ cup
Pear	1 small or ½ large
Plum	2

| Raspberries | 1 cup |
| Strawberries | 1 ¼ cup |

100% Fruit Juice · 1 serving

(Make sure label says 100% juice)

Apple juice	½ cup
Grapefruit juice	½ cup
Orange juice	½ cup
Pineapple juice	½ cup
Peach juice	½ cup
Pear juice	½ cup

Milk: Each serving of milk or milk product contains about 12 grams of carbohydrates and 8 grams of protein. Fat and calories vary, depending on what you select.

Skim and Very Low-fat Milk · 1 serving

| Skim—1% and 2% | 1 cup |
| Yogurt (low-fat or nonfat, no maltodextrins) | 6 oz. |

Fats and Oils: Each serving contains about 5 grams of fat and 45 calories. It is recommended that you eat mainly unsaturated fats.

Unsaturated Fats · 1 serving

Avocado	⅛ medium
Mayonnaise (diet)	1 Tbsp.
Nuts and seeds	
Almonds	6 whole
Cashews	1 Tbsp.
Pecans	2 whole
Peanuts	20 small or 10 large
Walnuts	2 whole
Other nuts	1 Tbsp.

Oil (corn, cottonseed, safflower, soybean, sunflower, olive, peanut)	1 tsp.
Olives	10 small or 5 large
Salad dressing (regular)	2 tsp.
Salad dressing (reduced calorie)	1 Tbsp.
Salad dressing (oil-based)	1 Tbsp.

Saturated Fats	**1 serving**
Butter	1 tsp.
Sour cream	2 Tbsp.
Cream cheese (lite)	1 Tbsp.

THE MEAL PLANS

Now that I've given you some basics on what to eat—glycemically acceptable foods—and what proportions in which to eat them, let's begin to put this information together to come up with some sample meal plans. To get you started, here is a list of meals covering a 7-day period.

SAMPLE MEAL PLANS
DAY 1

	2,000 cal.	1,800 cal.	1,650 cal.
Breakfast			
High Fiber Cereal	1 1/2 cups	1 1/2 cups	1 1/2 cups
or Whole Grain Bread	2 slices	2 slices	2 slices
Grapefruit	1 whole	1 whole	half
Skim Milk	8 oz.	8 oz.	8 oz.
Egg Whites	2	1	0
Acceptable Margarine	1 tsp.	1 tsp.	1 tsp.
Morning Snack			
Soy Food Product	1/2 serving	1/2 serving	1/2 serving
Unsweetened Orange Juice	8 oz.	8 oz.	8 oz.
Stone Wheat Crackers	6	6	6
Lunch			
Dry Whole Meal or Protein Pasta	1 cup	1 cup	1 cup
Broccoli/Spinach	1 cup	1 cup	1/2 cup
Grilled Chicken	3 oz.	3 oz.	2 oz.
Olive, Flax, Canola, or Peanut Oil	2 tsp.	1 tsp.	1 tsp.
Afternoon Snack			
Medium Apple	1	1	1
Pure Protein Bar	2/3 bar	1/2 bar	1/3 bar
Dinner			
Basmati or Brown Rice	2/3 cup	2/3 cup	2/3 cup
Green Beans	1 cup	1 cup	1 cup
Grilled Halibut	3 oz.	3 oz.	3 oz.
Acceptable Salad Dressing	2 tsp.	2 tsp.	2 tsp.
Salad (spinach, romaine, iceberg)	2 cup	2 cup	2 cup
Nighttime Snack			
Skim Milk	8 oz. milk	8 oz. milk	8 oz. milk
Soy Food Product (mix)	1/2 serving	1/2 serving	1/2 serving

DAY 2

	2,000 cal.	1,800 cal.	1,650 cal.
Breakfast			
Pumpernickel, toasted	2 slices	2 slices	2 slices
Alpine Lace Cheese	1 oz.	0	0
Blueberries	¾ cup	¾ cup	¾ cup
Dannon Lite Fruit Yogurt	6 oz.	6 oz.	6 oz.
Smart Balance Soft Spread	1 tsp.	1 tsp.	1 tsp.
Morning Snack			
Soy Protein Powder	½ serving	½ serving	½ serving
Apple Juice	8 oz.	8 oz.	8 oz.
Soda Crackers	8	4	4
Lunch			
Grilled Tuna	3 oz.	3 oz.	2 oz.
Asparagus	1 cup	1 cup	1 cup
Olive or Flaxseed Oil	2 tsp.	1 tsp.	1 tsp.
Cooked Barley	1 cup	1 cup	⅔ cup
Afternoon Snack			
Green Banana	1	1	½
Dinner			
Pork Tenderloin	3 oz.	3 oz.	3 oz.
Sweet Potato	1 large	1 large	1 large
Steamed Cauliflower	1 cup	1 cup	1 cup
Acceptable Oil-based Dressing	2 tsp.	2 tsp.	2 tsp.
Salad (spinach, romaine, iceberg)	2 cup	2 cup	2 cup
Nighttime Snack			
Skim Milk	8 oz. milk	8 oz. milk	8 oz. milk
Soy Food Product (mix)	½ serving	½ serving	½ serving

DAY 3

	2,000 cal.	1,800 cal.	1,650 cal.
Breakfast			
Special K Cereal	1 ½ cups	1 ½ cups	1 ½ cups
Skim Milk	1 cup	1 cup	1 cup
Strawberries	1 ¼ cup	1 ¼ cup	1 ¼ cup
Morning Snack			
9-grain Bread	2 slices	2 slices	2 slices
No-sugar Peanut Butter	1 Tbsp.	0	0
Smart Balance Soft Spread	1 tsp.	1 tsp.	1 tsp.
Plum	2 small	2 small	2 small
Lunch			
Wheat Tortillas	2	2	2
Grilled Chicken	3 oz.	3 oz.	2 oz.
Olive or Flaxseed Oil	2 tsp.	1 tsp.	1tsp.
Yellow, Red, Green Pepper			
Tomato, Onion (diced and mixed)	1 cup	1 cup	1 cup
Afternoon Snack			
Orange Juice	1 cup	1 cup	½ cup
Protein Powder	½ serving	½ serving	½ serving
Dinner			
Black Beans	1 cup	⅔ cup	⅔ cup
Lean Sirloin	3 oz.	3 oz.	3 oz.
Grilled Eggplant	1 cup	1 cup	1 cup
Acceptable Dressing	2 tsp.	2 tsp.	2 tsp.
Salad (spinach, romaine, iceberg)	2 cup	2 cup	2 cup
Nighttime Snack			
Skim Milk	8 oz. milk	8 oz. milk	8 oz. milk
Soy Food Product (mix)	½ serving	½ serving	½ serving
Medium Tangerine	1	1	1

DAY 4

	2,000 cal.	1,800 cal.	1,650 cal.
Breakfast			
Oat Bran Bread	2 slices	2 slices	2 slices
Canteloupe	1 cup	1 cup	1 cup
Skim Milk	1 cup	1 cup	1 cup
Morningstar Farms Sausage			
Breakfast Links	2 links	0	0
Acceptable Soft Spread	1 tsp.	1 tsp.	1 tsp.
Morning Snack			
Cottage Cheese, Lite	¼ cup	¼ cup	¼ cup
Stoned Wheat Crackers	6	6	6
Grapes	30	30	30
Lunch			
Gardenburger Soy Burger	1	1	1
Alpine Lace Cheese	1	1	1
Cracked Wheat Bun	1	1	1
Grilled Zucchini and Squash (mixed)	1 cup	1 cup	½ cup
Salad with Olive Oil	2 tsp.	1 tsp.	1 tsp.
Afternoon Snack			
Orange Juice	1 cup	1 cup	½ cup
Protein Powder	½ serving	½ serving	½ serving
Dinner			
Chinese Chicken	3 oz.	3 oz.	3 oz.
Broccoli	1 cup	1 cup	1 cup
Basmati Brown Rice	1 cup	1 cup	⅔ cup
Peanuts	2 oz.	2 oz.	2 oz.
Nighttime Snack			
Skim Milk	8 oz. milk	8 oz. milk	8 oz. milk
Soy Food Product (mix)	½ serving	½ serving	½ serving

DAY 5

Breakfast	2,000 cal.	1,800 cal.	1,650 cal.
Hot Bulgar Cereal	1 cup	1 cup	⅔ cup
Dannon Lite Fruit Yogurt	6 oz.	6 oz.	6 oz.
Raspberries	1 cup	1 cup	1 cup
Morning Snack			
Oat Bran Bread	1 slice	1 slice	1 slice
Alpine Lace Cheese	1 oz.	0	0
Grapefruit Juice	1 cup	1 cup	½ cup
Acceptable Spread	1 tsp.	1 tsp.	1 tsp.
Lunch			
Turkey, Sliced	3 oz.	3 oz.	2 oz.
Rye Toast	2 slices	2 slices	2 slices
Hellman's Lite Mayonnaise	2 tsp.	1 tsp.	1 tsp.
Acceptable Vegetables, Raw	1 cup	1 cup	1 cup
Stoned Wheat Crackers	6	0	0
Afternoon Snack			
Grapefruit Juice	1 cup	1 cup	1 cup
Protein Powder	½ serving	½ serving	½ serving
Dinner			
Macaroni	1 cup	1 cup	1 cup
Diced Chicken Breast	3 oz.	3 oz.	3 oz.
Green Beans and Mushrooms (mixed)	1 cup	1 cup	1 cup
Acceptable Dressing	2 tsp.	2 tsp.	2 tsp.
Salad (spinach, romaine, iceberg)	2 cup	2 cup	2 cup
Nighttime Snack			
Skim Milk	8 oz. milk	8 oz. milk	8 oz. milk
Soy Food Product (mix)	½ serving	½ serving	½ serving

DAY 6

	2,000 cal.	1,800 cal.	1,650 cal.
Breakfast			
High Fiber Cereal	1¾ cups	¾ cup	¾ cup
Skim Milk	1 cup	1 cup	1 cup
Strawberries	1¼ cups	1¼ cups	1¼ cups
Rye Toast	1 slice	0	0
Acceptable Fat	1 tsp.	0	0
Morning Snack			
Soy Protein Powder	½ serving	½ serving	½ serving
Orange Juice	1 cup	1 cup	½ cup
Soda Crackers	4	4	4
Lunch			
Vegetarian Hot Dog	1	1	1
Alpine Lace Cheese	1 slice	1 slice	0
Cracked Oat Bun	1	1	1
Acceptable Dressing	2 tsp.	1 tsp.	1 tsp.
Salad (spinach, romaine, iceberg)	2 cup	2 cup	2 cup
Soda Crackers	4	4	4
Afternoon Snack			
Cottage Cheese	½ cup	¼ cup	¼ cup
Large Apple	1	1	1
Dinner			
Lean Ham	3 oz.	3 oz.	3 oz.
Fettucine	1 cup	1 cup	1 cup
Stewed Okra and Tomatoes (mixed)	1 cup	1 cup	1 cup
Olive Oil	2 tsp.	2 tsp.	2 tsp.
Nighttime Snack			
Skim Milk	8 oz. milk	8 oz. milk	8 oz. milk
Soy Food Product (mix)	½ serving	½ serving	½ serving

DAY 7

	2,000 cal.	1,800 cal.	1,650 cal.
Breakfast			
Oatmeal	1 ½ cups	1 ½ cups	1 ½ cups
Skim Milk	1 cup	1 cup	1 cup
Medium Peach	1	1	1
Acceptable Spread	1 tsp.	1 tsp.	1 tsp.
Morning Snack			
Pineapple Juice	1 cup	1 cup	1 cup
Rye Toast	2 slices	2 slices	2 slices
Alpine Lace Cheese	1 slice	1 slice	1 slice
Lunch			
Tuna, Canned in Water	3 oz.	3 oz.	2 oz.
Stoned Wheat Crackers	12	12	12
Acceptable Dressing	2 tsp.	1 tsp.	1 tsp.
Salad (spinach, romaine, iceberg)	2 cups	2 cups	2 cups
Afternoon Snack			
Apple Juice	½ cup	½ cup	½ cup
Protein Powder	½ serving	½ serving	½ serving
Dinner			
Grilled Salmon	3 oz.	3 oz.	3 oz.
Large Sweet Potato	1	1	1
Cabbage/Spinach	1 cup	1 cup	1 cup
Acceptable Dressing	2 tsp.	2 tsp.	2 tsp.
Salad (spinach, romaine, iceberg)	2 cups	2 cups	2 cups
Nighttime Snack			
Skim Milk	8 oz. milk	8 oz. milk	8 oz. milk
Soy Food Product (mix)	½ serving	½ serving	½ serving

CHART YOUR OWN DAILY MEAL PLAN

Now that you've had a chance to see what seven days of meals looks like, you can begin to chart your own meal plans. Using the sample meals as a guide, and the list of glycemically acceptable foods, plan some new menus that meet your caloric needs. To make your job easier, I have included a meal-plan chart that you can photocopy and fill in.

DAILY MEAL PLAN CHART
55% low-glycemic carbohydrates, 25% lean meats, 20% acceptable fats

Breakfast
- Starch _____
- Meat _____
- Vegetable _____
- Fruit_____
- Milk _____
- Fat_____

Morning Snack _____
_____
_____

Lunch
- Starch _____
- Meat _____
- Vegetable _____
- Fruit_____
- Milk _____
- Fat_____

Afternoon Snack _____
_____
_____

Dinner
- Starch _____
- Meat _____
- Vegetable _____
- Fruit_____
- Milk _____
- Fat_____

Nighttime Snack _____
_____
_____

Breakfast
- Starch _____
- Meat _____
- Vegetable _____
- Fruit_____
- Milk _____
- Fat_____

Morning Snack _____
_____
_____

Lunch
- Starch _____
- Meat _____
- Vegetable _____
- Fruit_____
- Milk _____
- Fat_____

Afternoon Snack _____
_____
_____

Dinner
- Starch _____
- Meat _____
- Vegetable _____
- Fruit_____
- Milk _____
- Fat_____

Nighttime Snack _____
_____
_____

If you follow this food plan, eating low-glycemic foods in the right proportions, I guarantee that you will never feel hungry, you will have plenty of energy, and you will start seeing the inches melt off those love handles.

CHAPTER NOTES

[1] My thanks to Dr. Ann de Wees Allen and the Glycemic Research Institute for the following lists of acceptable and unacceptable glycemic foods, listed by category and name brand. Since this list is continually being updated and expanded, you can get further information by contacting the Glycemic Research Institute.

[2] The source of this information was the book *Glycemic Rating of Foods*, a booklet published by the Glycemic Research Institute, 601 Pennsylvania Avenue, NW, Ste. 900, Washington, D.C. 20004, (202) 434-8270.

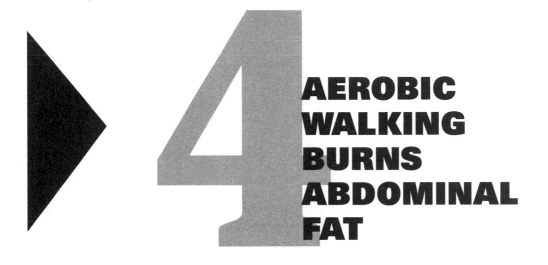

4 AEROBIC WALKING BURNS ABDOMINAL FAT

By now you are probably getting the picture that no one is born fat. We become overweight through poor diet and lack of activity. While it is true that 50 percent of our body composition comes from our genetic heritage and our childhood eating habits, the other 50 percent comes from the choices we make at the dinner table and how much of a workout we give our bodies every day.

WALKING IS A BIG HEALTH PLUS

The first step toward becoming more physically active is aerobic walking. Walking between 45 and 60 minutes a day is by far one of the easiest and most beneficial forms of exercise that anyone can engage in. And the health benefits are considerable. A recent article published by the American College of Sports Medicine states that aerobic activity reduces insulin resistance in people who suffer from obesity. This study also showed that aerobic training reduces fat mass without changing fat-free mass. In other words, if you want to lose more fat versus lean muscle, aerobic exercise is the ticket. Another study published in the *Medical Tribune* that was conducted on 2,678 men between the ages of 71 and 93 found that the risk of developing heart disease decreased 15 percent for every half mile walked per day. This is incredible news for two reasons. One is that if you walk two miles per day, you've decreased your risk for coronary disease by over 50 percent. The other is that it is clearly *never* too late to start walking and to derive benefits from it. In fact, as you age, it actually takes less effort to achieve a training effect on your cardiovascular system.

STARTING YOUR AEROBIC WALKING PROGRAM

The great thing about walking is that it doesn't take any special equipment other than a good pair of walking or running shoes, and it can be done anywhere, whether you live in the city, town, or country. Walking is also easy on the joints. Remember, before you embark on this or any other exercise program, be sure to check with your physician.

When buying a pair of walking shoes, I suggest that you shop at a store that specializes in sports footwear. Not only will you find a wide range of brands and prices, you will have the benefit of an experienced salesperson to help you find the shoe that's best for you. Explaining to the salesperson where you plan to walk (city sidewalks, on a treadmill in a gym, on a track, up and down hills, along the beach) will enable him or her to suggest the most appropriate footwear. The kind of shoe you would wear walking on city sidewalks is quite different from the kind of shoe you would wear walking on the uneven terrain of a woodland hiking trail. You should also be aware of what your personal idiosyncrasies are. If you have a tendency to roll toward the inside of your foot when you walk, then you should probably look for a well-padded shoe that is built for control and stability. If you roll your weight toward the outsides of your feet, try a shoe that has firm heel support and good shock absorbency under the ball of the foot. Taking a look at your old shoes should give you a general idea of your walking pattern. Make sure that you take your time and really walk around in the store while wearing the shoes before you buy them. If you are shopping in a store that has incline ramps in the shoe department, try walking in place facing down the ramp to make sure your toes will not be banging against the front of your shoe on a hill. Avoid the smaller possible size, and allow for some extra room at your toes. Always shop in the latter part of the day, after your feet have had a chance to swell. A shoe that feels terrific at 10:00 in the morning may feel uncomfortably tight after 3:00 P.M.

Do not buy shoes because they are a certain brand name or because somebody else told you how great they are. Try on several brands before making your final decision. Buy the ones that fit your feet best. Not all feet are the same and not all shoe companies make shoes for the same feet. Some companies make their shoes with high arches, others with low arches, and others make theirs for wide feet; others make their shoes for narrow feet. Keep in mind that most of the activities we do, especially walking, start at the feet. It is important that we provide our feet with the best environment possible. Also remember to invest in some good pairs of thick socks made from natural fibers such as cotton or soft wool.

When walking, it is best to wear comfortable, loose, lightweight clothes. Wear natural fibers such as cotton to allow the body's heat to escape during the warm months of the year. Don't forget your sunscreen if you are walking before 4:30 P.M. It may not seem that you could get much sun walking for 45 to 60 minutes six times a week, but if you are fair-skinned and not used to being outside during the day, you could easily get too much sun. You will probably be more comfortable in exercise clothing that is made of "wicking" fibers that absorb moisture and keep you from feeling damp and clammy if you perspire a lot. In colder weather, it is best to dress in layers. This helps to hold in body heat and allows you to peel off layers as you warm up. On cold or rainy days it is important to wear a hat and gloves since much of your body heat is lost through those extremities.

Prior to walking allow for a brief 5 to 10 minute warm-up period, which will prepare your body for aerobic activity and help to reduce the chances of muscle strain. This could mean gently stretching the body before exercising or starting out by walking slowly and then increasing the pace.

Some tips on getting the most out of your aerobic walking include walking tall and watching your posture, taking even and comfortable strides, allowing your arms to swing in a relaxed and free way, and breathing in fully and exhaling fully.

If your goal is to walk, say, two miles a day, how can you determine the distance? If you are walking on a treadmill in the gym, the settings will tell you when you have walked the equivalent of one mile. If you know that it takes you 20 minutes to walk a mile on the treadmill, you can pretty much estimate by looking at landmarks how much a mile is on even terrain out of doors. Or you can use the odometer in your car to determine the distance or map out a route. If you are walking in the city, you might want to buy a pedometer.

HOW TO MAXIMIZE FAT BURNING DURING AEROBIC EXERCISE

The body's ability to select and burn body fat during exercise is dependent on two elements: what you put into your body just prior to exercise and the intensity and duration of the exercise. Taking simple sugars such as juice or candy prior to exercise can cause the body to temporarily emphasize glucose (blood sugar) as its main energy source. This abundant sugar in your bloodstream is going to minimize your body's ability to reach into your fat stores and burn them for energy. Taking in simple sugars might make you subject to reactive hypoglycemia—low blood sugar due to your insulin response, which will compromise the duration and quality of your aerobic steady-state training. In other words, your blood sugar will take a big jump upward and then take a plunge downward, leaving you feeling suddenly tired. It is far better to not eat anything just before a walk unless you are a diabetic, in which case you should consult your doctor.

When at rest, your body releases adipose fat tissue at a rate of about 50 percent fat, 50 percent glucose. Walking at a steady-state comfortable pace causes you to utilize 40 percent of your oxygen consumption. At this steady-state rate of walking, your body will eventually shift its source of energy until it is taking almost 85 percent from fat storage. As your body begins speeding up its rate of releasing fatty acids (triglycerides) from adipose fat tissue, your muscles signal the brain to release more stored fat for fuel. It takes about 20 to 30 minutes for your body to get the signal and go into full fat-release mode. That is why I suggest that you make each of your aerobic walking sessions at least 45 to 60 minutes long. Obviously, if some days you can walk more than that, you will increase your benefits.

It is possible to walk too fast, however. An easy way to make sure that you are not walking too fast to take advantage of the maximum fat-burning zone is the "talk test." This test was developed by Bill Bowerman, a highly respected former track coach. If you can carry on a conversation with yourself or a partner without huffing and puffing, then you will know that you are walking at a good pace. If you find that you get out of breath when you talk, you should slow down because you are actually causing the body to burn more carbohydrates than excess body fat as fuel. Walking at a conversational pace allows you to tap into inexhaustible fat stores and keep going for extended periods of time.

Another way to tell if you are exercising at the proper aerobic intensity—exerting yourself enough to get your heart pumping significantly above its rate at rest, yet still somewhat below its maximum—is to take the pulse test. Your ideal aerobic training goal is to have your heart beating at 75 percent of its maximum. You can measure whether or not you are in that zone in the following way.

Measuring Your Training Rate
Using the Pulse Test

Step 1

To find your maximum heart rate,
subtract your age from 220.

Step 2

Multiply this number by 75 percent to find the middle range
of intensity for your aerobic exercise.

Step 3

In the morning, before you get out of bed, take your pulse
for a full 60 seconds. This is called your "resting pulse rate."
Use either wrist or the carotid artery in your neck.

Step 4

Immediately after exercising, take your pulse for 6 seconds
and multiply that number times 10. This is your "training pulse rate."
This number should not be more than the answer to Step 2. If it is
below that number, you need to exert yourself more. If it is above
that number, you should pull back a bit.

Be aware that certain medications or situations may cause fluctuations in the heart rate. For some individuals, this formula may over- or underestimate the maximum heart rate. Check with your physician concerning your maximum heart rate.

Eventually, you will be able to take up to 90 percent of the total energy utilized during low-to-moderate intensity exercise from the stores of fat in your body. For this reason, as you practice your aerobic walking over time and with consistency, it will help your body get very good at burning fat.

Although some of the men in our study were not able to do so, it is better by far to do your walking 1½ hours before dinner, when your daily metabolism is lowest, because that will increase your metabolism by up to 50 percent. Once you have hit your fat-burning zone, it takes 4 hours for pulse rate to return to normal. If your metabolism (burning of glucose) is elevated, whatever you eat will be used more quickly as fuel as opposed to being stored as fat.

Another benefit, as we have seen, is in the normalizing of insulin production. By curtailing insulin's effect on fat storage and enhancing glucogon effect on fat mobilization, you can teach your body to stop storing excess fat and start burning it for fuel during exercise.

The really good news is that if you are trying to lose weight in the love-handle area, low-to-moderate exercise such as aerobic walking gives fat in the core areas of the body, most especially abdominal fat, the preferential treatment, causing you to lose it even faster than you will be losing peripheral fat (fat on the outside of the body). Men are born with more fat cells in the abdominal area of the body and therefore will tend to store fat there before any other area. Walk down any street in America, and you will see dozens of men with big bellies and skinny legs. As men accumulate more and more fat through poor lifestyle habits, increasing stress, and declining testosterone levels (with age), the majority of fat keeps being deposited deep inside the abdomen. Since exercise causes the body to draw first on its preferential fat stores, abdominal fat is the first to be burned.

Just as you warm up before your aerobic walking, remember to allow yourself some time to cool down. One way to do this is by gradually decreasing your pace to allow your body to return to a resting state. Doing strength and flexibility exercises—or even some simple stretches—is another good way to cool down after walking.

Warning signs to watch for if you are overdoing your walking program might include:

- Severe shortness of breath.
- Wheezing or coughing.
- Chest pain or tightness in chest.

- Excessive perspiration.
- Dizziness or nausea.
- Severe muscle cramps or aches.
- Prolonged exhaustion after exercising.

If you experience any of these symptoms while walking, stop and rest for about 10 or 15 minutes. Call your doctor if these symptoms do not disappear after resting.

Some normal reactions to increased physical activity include:

- Faster but not uncomfortable heart rate.
- Quicker rate of breathing.
- Mild to moderate perspiring.
- Muscle soreness that might last a day or two at the start of your walking program.

WHEN AND HOW OFTEN YOU SHOULD WALK

I suggest walking six times a week for maximum effect. You could even walk daily because the benefits are so great and the wear and tear on the body are so minimal. The ideal time to walk is about 1½ hours before eating your evening meal because that will increase your metabolism at dinner time by 50 percent.

If you absolutely can't walk in the late afternoon or early evening because of your work schedule, it is better to walk at any time of the day than not at all. Some of the men who participated in my 30-day program did most of their aerobic walking in the early morning before work or on the treadmill in the gym before their morning workout.

Another benefit of walking before dinner, however, is that it gives you a chance to make a transition from your workday to your evening with friends and family. I myself often use this time to do a simple meditation exercise called Freeze Frame®, which is designed to reduce your daily stress level. While walking, pick a stressful event or personal relationship and make a snapshot of it in your mind. Next shift your attention from the racing thoughts in your brain by focusing your attention on your heart. It is helpful to imagine that you are breathing through your heart. Next, envision an enjoyable experience in your life or the most peaceful and beautiful setting you can imagine and recreate that image. For some of you, this might be an ocean beach, a trout stream, or your favorite place in the woods. For me, it is my wife and children and I in a family hug. Next, employing your common sense, intuition, and sincerity, use the link between your heart and your brain to envision a solution to the stressful personal relationship or event. Listen to how your heart responds to your question. You might be pleasantly surprised at what happens. If you practice this meditation over time, you will certainly learn to more effectively manage stress, develop more resources for problem solving, and notice benefits to your cardiovascular system and to your central nervous system.

Below is a walking chart to help you keep track of the time you spend doing this aerobic exercise. You may also wish to enter your daily mileage. Many of my clients find it helpful to keep track of what kind of terrain they walk on if they have different courses; whether or not they walk more often in a gym versus walking outside; what kind of elevation they walk on a particular day; or anything else that they find helpful.

AEROBIC WALKING CHART

Day	Mon.	Tues.	Wed.	Thurs.	Fri.	Sat.	Sun.
Week 1	Walked 45 min—felt great.						
Week 2							
Week 3							
Week 4							
Week 5							
Week 6							
Week 7							
Week 8							

FIGURE 4.1: AEROBIC WALKING CHART

WAYS TO STAY MOTIVATED

If you find that you are having trouble finding time for your walking program, it helps to give yourself reasons to keep motivated. I suggest the following strategies:

- Set specific and realistic goals. Initially, you may find it hard to walk 60 minutes, but feel good about walking 30. Try increasing your time by 5 minutes every 3 or 4 days until you can work your way up to 45, and then gradually increase to 60 minutes per day. If you are very obese, initially you might only be able to walk 10 or 15 minutes a day. There is nothing wrong with that. The important thing is to accomplish what you can and to gradually build up to 60 minutes when your body is truly ready to do so. Developing a consistent cardio-walking routine that you can gradually improve is far more important than doing more than you can handle in the beginning, feeling discouraged, and wanting to quit.
- Do something fun and entertaining when you walk. Go walking with your partner or a good friend, bring along your kids (if they are old enough to keep up with your optimum pace), or walk your dog. One man who did my program walked with his whole family before dinner. His wife and he would exchange news about the day while they walked, and the kids would ride their bikes back and forth. If you like to enjoy your favorite CD on a Discman while you walk outside, just make sure that the music is not so loud that you zone out to what is going on around you. Pay attention to traffic and to other potential dangers in your environment.
- Use your walking time to run an errand or to do something practical. Instead of falling into the habit of driving everywhere, walk instead.
- Walk in an interesting place. While walking in the gym may be ideal for some, others may want to vary the places where they walk. Intersperse walking in your local park with walking on a beautiful woodland trail on the weekends. Vary walking along the beach with walking around your neighborhood. If you live in a city like New York or Boston, plan your walk so that you pass through interesting ethnic neighborhoods or a beautiful part of town. Another great place to walk is in your local mall, which provides interesting things to look at and a comfortable

temperature regardless of the time of year. The world is full of great places to walk, and the possibilities are endless.

■ If you achieve your goals and remain consistent with your walking plan, give yourself a reward. Treating yourself to a pepperoni pizza and a hunk of chocolate cake is not a good idea. But buying season tickets to your favorite sporting event, going away for the weekend to a local vacation spot, or getting yourself or your family something you've been wanting are all ways of thanking yourself for accomplishing your goals.

TROUBLESHOOTING

If you find yourself developing aches and pains, take an inventory on what you are doing. Do you have inadequate footwear or shoes that have worn out? Are you walking up hilly terrain without proper physical preparation? Is your downhill walk out of control? More injuries occur when walking downhill. Do you allow yourself enough of a warm-up and cooldown? Are you drinking enough water to keep yourself hydrated? On hot, muggy days, it's always a good idea to carry a water bottle with you. I recommend keeping a bottle of water with you anytime you exercise and to drink from it regularly.

MOVING ON

If, over time, you want to move beyond this aerobic walking program, you may try some more intense exercises, such as jogging, using the stair machine, or swimming, as long as you adhere to the rules of the game.

One aerobic workout that is a logical extension of walking is racewalking. The benefits include an even more vigorous cardiovascular workout and even quicker weight loss. The talk test applies to racewalking as well. Having the proper kind of shoes is especially important in racewalking, as is making sure that you give yourself a chance to warm up. Some simple tips include:

■ Maintaining the correct posture. Allow your body to lean forward slightly, keeping your weight on the balls of your feet. Make sure your shoulders are relaxed and your back is comfortably straight.

- While keeping your shoulders straight, move your hips back and forth to increase the length of your stride.
- Hold your arms close to your body, keeping your fingers in a loose fist. You can swing your hands forward as high as your nipple line, but don't allow your elbows to swing out.
- Always keep one foot in contact with the ground.
- Keep your head relaxed and aligned with the rest of your body, ears over the shoulders. Watch out for side-to-side motion.
- Keep your eyes focused 20 to 30 feet ahead of you. [See Figure 4.2, Racewalking Posture]

Added to the low-glycemic meal plan, this aerobic walking program will have a tremendous affect on reducing fat in your abdominal area. So, get busy walking off those unwanted inches and getting your life back on track.

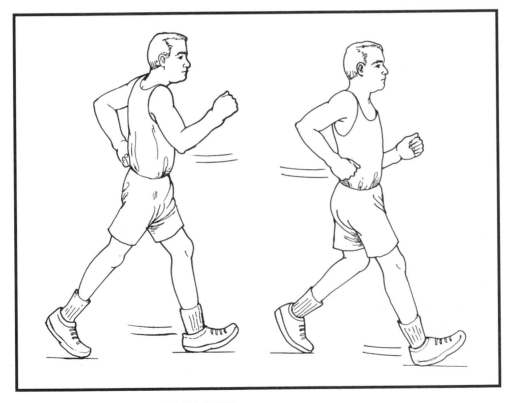

FIGURE 4.2, RACEWALKING POSTURE

CHAPTER NOTES

[1] The Freeze Frame meditation was developed by Doc Lew Childre in his book *Freeze Frame*. Childre is the president and CEO of the Institute of HeartMath, a nonprofit think tank specializing in innovative approaches to the problems of human stress, and to quality of life, creativity, and effectiveness.

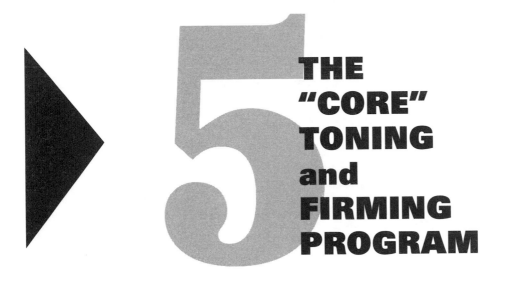

THE "CORE" TONING and FIRMING PROGRAM

The third element of my program for losing abdominal fat is my resistance exercise program for the core area of the body, which includes the spinal erectors, the abdominal muscles (rectus, transverse, and oblique), the gluteal muscles, the quadriceps, and the hamstrings. While people can lose weight by diet alone, exercise is key to keeping weight off. A recent article in the *International Journal of Obesity* described an 18-month study of a group of police officers who participated in an 8-week diet plus exercise program, which included 35 to 60 minutes of aerobic activity, calisthenics, and relaxation techniques three days per week. Those who did not keep exercising at the end of the study had gained back 60 percent of the weight lost at the end of a 6-month period, and 97 percent of their weight loss at the end of 18 months. These figures are consistent with many other studies that I've read and certainly with my own experiences working with many hundreds of athletes and laypeople over the last 25 years.

Exercise also determines what *kind* of weight you will lose, and how fast you will lose it. As I've said below, losing pounds of scale weight is less important to our general health and longevity than losing body fat. Dieting alone often leads to short-term weight loss, lowered metabolic rate, and loss of muscle mass, which makes us age more quickly. Dieting plus exercise is guaranteed to increase your lean-muscle to fat ratio and your metabolic rate and decrease your resistance to insulin. In a properly prescribed program like this one, the goal is to preserve lean body tissue at the expense of body fat.

When starting an exercise program, it is important not to be discouraged if the inches don't melt off right away. Whether or not you see yourself shrinking over the short term, you will certainly lose both weight and waistline inches over the long term. And you can be assured that, from day one, your body is receiving a multitude of benefits from these core resistance exercises. One 6-month study conducted on individuals who were severely obese showed dramatic health benefits from proper nutrition and exercise performed four to five times per week. Although these individuals were still rated in the obese category at the end of this period, their serum cholesterols, triglycerides, blood pressures, and resting heart rates had all dropped from the abnormally high range into the normal range.

Exercise also helps us to manage insulin. People who suffer from type 1 or type 2 diabetes, or are at risk for developing these conditions, can benefit from making regular exercise a part of their lifestyle. Studies at the University of California found following the benefits of regular exercise:

- Improved glucose tolerance through enhancing insulin sensitivity.
- Helped individuals to either lose weight or to maintain their ideal weight because of the increase in their metabolic rate.
- Enabled some individuals to either take less medication, or to stop taking medication altogether.
- Improved energy level, strength, flexibility, quality of life, and general sense of well being.

The exercises in this chapter are designed not to work the entire body, but to tone, firm, and stabilize the all-important core area. If you want to get an entire-body workout, I suggest that you combine my program with some circuit or weight training at your local gym or YMCA. [SEE FIGURE 5.1]

It is always a good idea to check with your health care provider before starting an exercise program if you are:

- Over forty.
- Overweight.
- Have a history of cardiac disease.
- Have orthopedic problems or a chronic medical condition.

If you are obese or have not exercised for a long period of time, I suggest that you begin slowly. I have provided two different programs for you to choose from. You should do each one in its entirety, at least four times per week. Once this program has become routine, you should be able to do it in 15 to 20 minutes. When that happens, I suggest that you try and do the exercises six to seven times per week. Although the second program is more advanced, each includes core resistance exercises that are designed to stabilize the upper pelvis, lower pelvis, and the upper torso. Even though you will lose both weight and inches on this program, and build a powerful core area, I encourage you to consult a trainer about enhancing your benefits by adding weight training or resistance exercises for other parts of your body, such as your arms.

You will notice that one of the programs includes the use of Swiss balls, which have become very popular in athletic training. Your gym or health spa will certainly have balls available for use. If you wish to purchase your

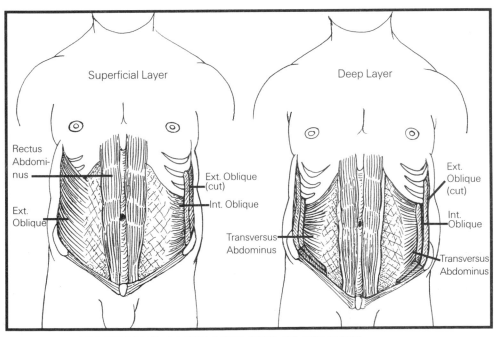

FIGURE 5.1 THE MUSCLES OF THE CORE AREA OF THE BODY.

own ball, you may do so at most sporting goods stores, where they are reasonably priced, or you can contact CDM Medical, a mail-order company that sells Swiss balls and medicine balls. Their contact numbers are 800-400-7542 (office), 817-448-8701 (FAX), and Web site: www.cdmsports.com.

For most exercises, the size ball you need is one that allows your thighs to be raised slightly above the horizontal when you are seated on it. (See photographs of exercises on page 112.) One method of deciding which diameter ball you need is to take your body height in centimeters and subtract 100 from that figure. Or you can try out a few size balls and see which one feels best to you.

Swiss balls are an effective training tool for increasing strength, improving body stability, and increasing the stability and flexibility of joints. The slight instability of the ball increases the body's ability to balance and stabilize itself. When using the balls, it is helpful to exercise in front of a mirror so that you can monitor your body position. But if you do not have access to Swiss balls or other equipment, the Core Exercise Program, Routine I, can be done at home easily and safely. You may wish to try both Routine I and Routine II to see which one feels best on your body, but you should ultimately pick one program and stick to it.

I have put together a chart for you that shows the proper order in which to do Routine 1 and Routine 2, and suggests the number of repetitions you should start with and your optimum goals. For most exercises, I suggest you start out with something that feels comfortable to you, like 1 set of 10 repetitions, and build up to 2 sets of 25. If 1 set of 10 seems like too much in the beginning, do less. And never continue an exercise if you feel any discomfort. Stop, readjust your position, look at your form, and try again. Should the discomfort continue, consult with a personal trainer or a physical therapist for the proper technique. If you have had a history of back problems, or surgery in the core area of the body, I recommend that you consult with your doctor before beginning this program.

Although it is possible to do each of these routines in as little as 15 to 20 minutes, don't expect to be able to do that at first. As with all exercise programs, there is a learning curve involved. Eventually, as you build up strength, you will be able to do more repetitions in less time—and do the exercises 6 to 7 times per week. The important thing to remember is to not give up and to be consistent. I guarantee that, even if these exercises seem a bit tough at first, your body will get used to them. The six men who spent 14 weeks in this program prior to the writing of this book all admitted that it took them a little while to really get into the routines. But once they did, they all spoke enthusiastically about how strong they felt, how much better they were managing their daily stress, and the positive feedback they were getting about their appearance from family, colleagues, and friends.

I have also included a routine for preexercise warm up and postexercise cooldown. If you do not belong to a gym, where this stretch device is readily available, you can either buy it at your local sporting goods store or order tubing from DKSA, 800-217-5282 (office), 802-362-0825 (FAX), Web site: www.stretchout.com.

Wear comfortable, lightweight clothing. You will be more comfortable—at home or at a gym—working on a mat or other padded surface.

Stretch Strap Routine

Perform all stretches with one leg, then repeat with the other leg.
Hold all stretches 2–5 seconds. Don't bounce. Keep a steady tension on strap.
Your Goal: Use this routine to warm up and cooldown.

Exercise 1:

Insert your foot into the strap and lift your leg. Lock one end of the strap around your heel and the other end around your ankle. Place the loop of the strap around your neck and shoulder. Grasp the strap with one hand as shown and pull your foot toward the opposite shoulder.

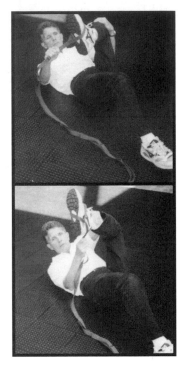

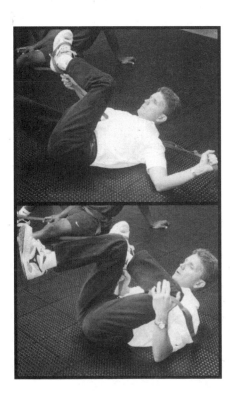

Exercise 2:

Return foot to starting position. Bring the opposite knee to your chin while pulling the strapped leg toward your chest.

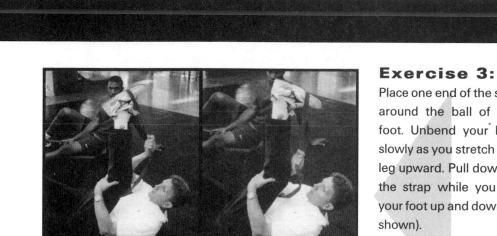

Exercise 3:

Place one end of the strap around the ball of your foot. Unbend your knee slowly as you stretch your leg upward. Pull down on the strap while you flex your foot up and down (as shown).

Exercise 4:

First, place one end of the strap around your heel and use the strap (as shown) to pull your outstretched leg to the opposite shoulder as far as you can comfortably reach. Swing your leg back and switch the strap to the opposite heel. Swing your leg directly over your torso and bring the outstretched leg as close as possible to your forehead while pulling the strap directly overhead (as shown).

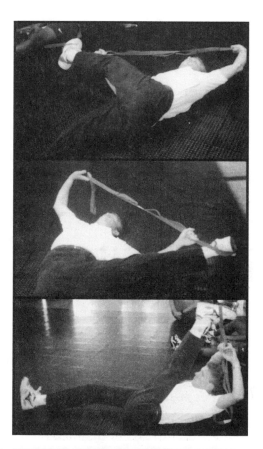

Stretch Strap Routine

Exercise 5:

Turn onto your side so that your unstrapped leg is resting on the floor. Keep the strap in position around your heel. Grasping the strap behind your head, pull your leg upward. Do not bend your knee more than 90 degrees. Feel the stretch in your hip.

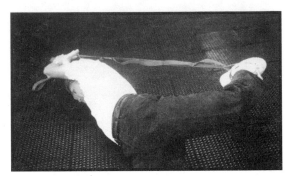

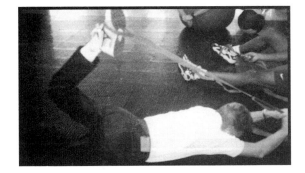

Exercise 6:

Roll onto your stomach while keeping the tension on the strap. Continue pulling the strap from overhead (as shown). Again, stretch from the hip, but do not bend the knee more than 90 degrees.

Repeat all exercises with your other leg. When you have finished with your Core Exercise Program, repeat the Stretch Strap Routine to cooldown.

Core Exercise Program

Core Exercises

- ► Standard Crunch
- ► Reverse Crunch
- ► Oblique Crunch
- ► Reverse Trunk Twist
- ► Bridge
- ► Superman
- ► Cross Body Lift
- ► Back Raises
- ► Side Twists
- ► Cat Stretch

Start with 1 set of 10 and work up to 25 repetitions performed 6 to 7 times per week. Your emphasis should be on doing one complete circuit of core exercises and rotational exercises, using the same number of repetitions for each exercise. Gradually increase your repetitions. The emphasis should be on maintaining your form at all times.

Rotational Routine

- ► Wood Chopping
- ► Standing Russian Twists
- ► Discus Throw

Use a light medicine ball (2–3 lbs.) or clasp your hands together. Start with 1 set of 10 and work up to 25 repetitions, using the same number of repetitions for each exercise. Gradually increase your repetitions. The emphasis should be on maintaining your form at all times.

Your Goal: Do the entire Core Exercise Program in the A.M. and 45–60 minutes of walking in the P.M.

Exercise Routine 1: Floor

Standard Crunch (Upper Abdominals):

Lie on your back with your head on the floor and your arms crossed over your chest, legs bent and feet flat on the floor. Raise your head and shoulders off the ground. Hold for a few seconds, then lower your head and shoulders to the starting position.

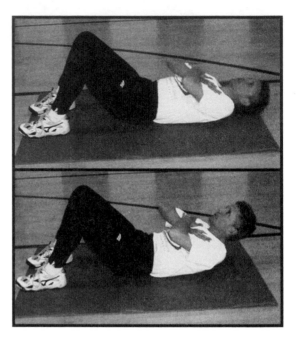

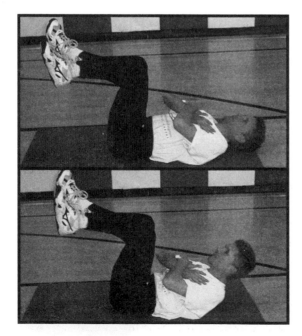

Standard Crunch— Advanced (Upper Abdominals):

Lie on your back with your head on the floor and your arms crossed over your chest, and your legs bent and lifted off the floor. Cross your ankles. Raise your head and shoulders off the ground. Hold for a few seconds, then lower your head and shoulders to the starting position.

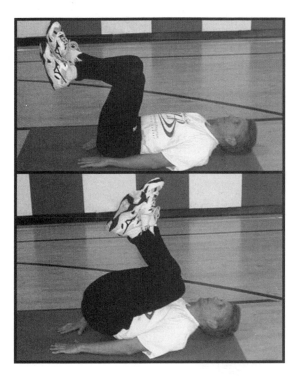

Reverse Crunch
(Lower Abdominals):

Lie on your back with your head on the floor, arms braced at your sides with palms on the floor. Legs are raised and knees bent at a right angle with calves parallel to the floor. Cross your ankles. Begin by bringing your legs back toward your chest while contracting your lower abs. Slowly move back to the starting position.

Oblique Crunch:

Lie flat on your back with left foot flat on the floor. Cross the ankle of your right foot over your lower thigh. Place the left hand to the side of your head, elbow out, and extend your other arm perpendicular to your side, palm down. Begin by curling your upper body forward at the waist. Contract your torso across your midsection and try to touch your elbow to your knee (as shown). Squeeze your elbow to your knee. Lower your body to the floor. Switch legs and arms and repeat.

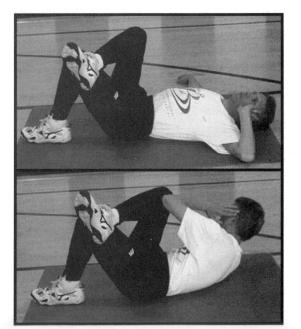

Exercise Routine 1: Floor

Reverse Trunk Twist:

Lie faceup on the floor with your arms out to the sides, palms down, and your legs in the air, knees bent at a right angle, with calves parallel to the floor. Cross your ankles. Contract your abs and lower your legs to one side, exhaling and keeping your knees together. Touch the floor with your legs while keeping your shoulders and arms in full contact with the floor. Inhale and raise your legs back to the starting position. Without stopping, continue over to the opposite side until your legs touch the floor again. Exhale as you lower your legs. Continue alternating. One repetition includes both sides. Note: Try and keep your shoulders in contact with the floor at all times.

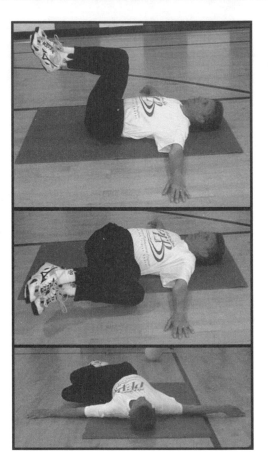

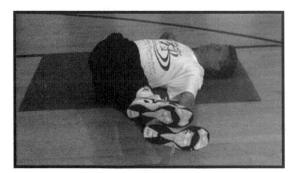

Advanced Version of Reverse Trunk Twist:

When you have gained strength, you can perform this exercise with your legs extended.

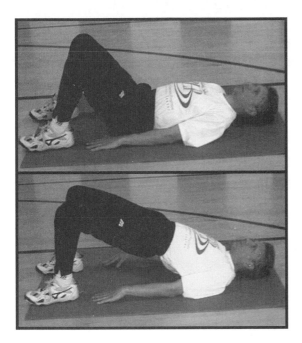

Bridge:

Lie faceup on the floor with your arms by your side, palms down, feet flat on the floor with your knees bent. Tighten your abs and raise your trunk until your body forms a straight line between your knees and your shoulders. Slowly lower yourself to the starting position.

Superman:

Lie facedown on the floor with a 6–8-inch pillow (when compressed—a folded towel is another option) under your lower abdominal pelvic region. Raise your trunk, arms, and legs all at the same time so that your entire body is horizontal with the floor. Hold 2–3 seconds and relax.

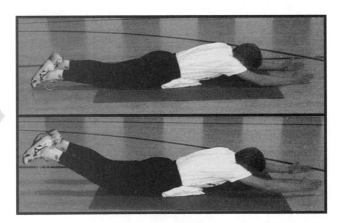

105

Exercise Routine 1: Floor

Superman (Alternating):

If you find the first version of this exercise difficult, you may want to try an easier variation. Perform this exercise raising alternate legs and arms (right arm and left leg, left arm and right leg). One repetition includes both sides.

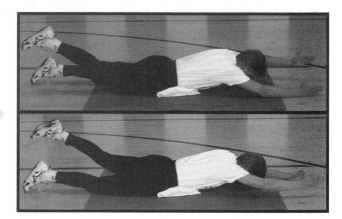

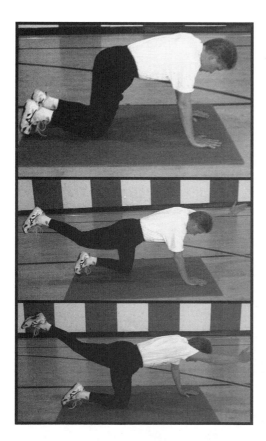

Cross Body Lift:

Get down on all fours with your back straight. Tighten your abdominal muscles and slowly raise one arm and its opposite leg until they are in line or slightly above the level of your back. Slowly return to the starting position and repeat on the opposite side.

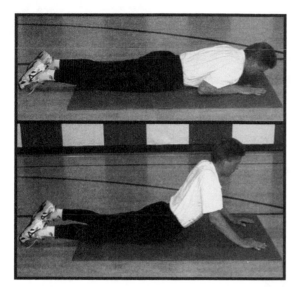

Back Raises:

Lie facedown on the floor with the legs together and the upper body slightly raised, supported on the forearms. Tighten your abs and raise your upper torso as far as you can without discomfort. Pause and flex the abdominal muscles for a few seconds, then lower yourself to the starting position.

Side Twists:

Lie on the floor on your back with your hands behind your head, feet flat on the floor, and knees bent. Keeping your shoulders on the floor, drop your knees to the right and touch them to the floor. Pause and flex your abdominal muscles for a few seconds. Then, in one continuous motion, raise your knees and drop them to the left. Exhale as you lower your legs and inhale as your raise them. One repetition includes both sides.

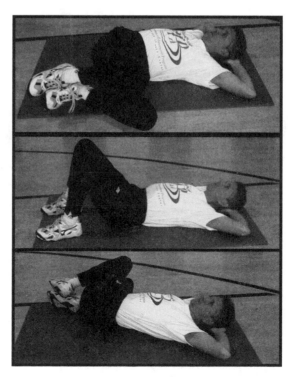

Exercise Routine 1: Floor

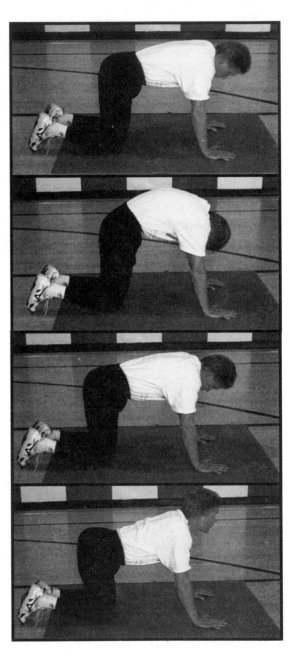

Cat Stretch:

Get down on all fours with your back straight and your hands and knees shoulder width apart. Begin by inhaling, then exhale as you pull your stomach to your spine, rounding your back upward and dropping your head until you are looking toward your pelvis. Feel this movement in your lower back. Lower your back, inhale as you pass through the neutral position, then exhale as you bring your head up, pulling your shoulders down as you feel your spine extend. Repeat in each direction three times.

Rotation Routine

Note: Use a 2–3 pound medicine ball to do these exercises. If you don't have a medicine ball, you can do these exercises with your hands clasped together.

Wood Chopping:

Stand with your knees slightly flexed, shoulder width apart, and your upper body erect. Hold the ball raised in front of you so the ball is above the level of your head. Swing the ball forward and downward in a chopping motion until it is between your legs. In one smooth motion, slowly return to the starting position. If you are using a medicine ball, make sure to always control the weight of the ball.

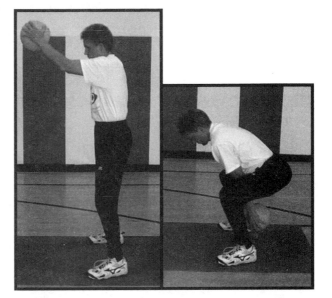

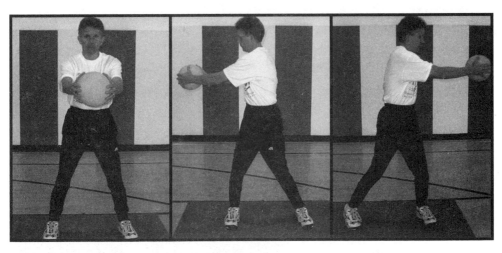

Standing Russian Twist:

Stand with your knees slightly flexed, shoulder width apart, and your upper body erect. Hold the ball out in front of you, arms extended, with the ball at waist level. Alternate between twisting to the left and twisting to the right. *Begin slowly* and only increase your speed after you have become familiar with the exercise. Always move in a controlled manner, especially if you are doing this exercise with a medicine ball.

Rotation Routine

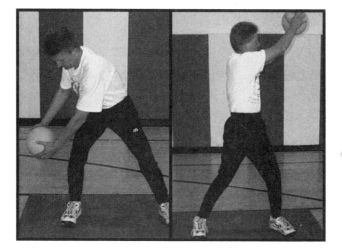

Discus Throw:

Stand with your knees flexed, shoulder width apart. With your arms extended, hold the ball no higher than the waist position. (See starting position for Standing Russian Twist.) Bending your knees and twisting your body to the right side, swing the ball down toward the level of your right knee. Swing the ball up above your opposite shoulder (as shown). Return to the neutral position and repeat on the opposite side. One repetition includes both sides. Always move in a controlled manner, especially if using a medicine ball.

Core Exercise Program

Core Exercises

- ▶ Bridge
- ▶ Upper Abdominal Crunch
- ▶ Upper Back Extension
- ▶ Lower Abdominal Crunch
- ▶ Double Leg Curl
- ▶ Hamstring Stretch
- ▶ Lower Extension
- ▶ Wall Squat

Seated on exercise ball. Start with 1 set of 10 and work up to 25 repetitions. Your emphasis should be on doing one complete circuit of core exercises and rotational exercises, using the same number of repetitions for each exercise. Gradually increase your repetitions. The emphasis should be on maintaining your form at all times.

Rotational Routine

- ▶ Chop
- ▶ Lift
- ▶ ½ Rotation

Seated on ball with chord. Start with one set of 10 and work up to 25 repetitions, using the same number of repetitions for each exercise. Gradually increase your repetitions. The emphasis should be on maintaining your form at all times.

Your Goal: Do the entire Core Exercise Program in the A.M., and 45–60 minutes of walking in the P.M.

The "Core" Toning and Firming Program

Core Exercise Routine 2: Ball Program

Bridge:

Sit on the floor with your upper back and neck resting on the ball with your feet flat on the floor. Lift your buttocks slightly up off the floor and stabilize the ball with your head and shoulders before lifting the body into a bridging position. Hold for 2–3 seconds, then slowly lower yourself down into the stabilized position. Do not touch the floor.

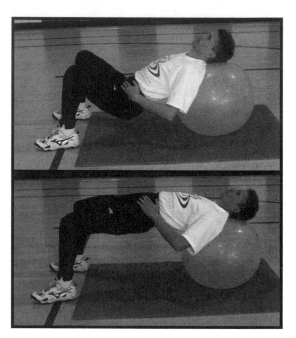

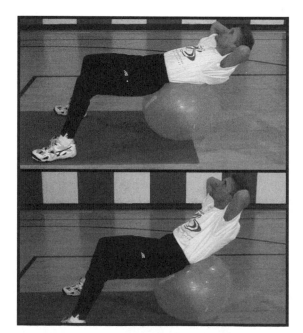

Upper Abdominal Crunch:

Lie on the ball with the middle of your back supported. Your feet should be flat on the floor, slightly wider apart than shoulder width. Clasp your hands behind your head with elbows out to the side and tighten your abs. Lift the upper part of your torso up off of the ball. Hold 2–3 seconds, then slowly return to the starting position.

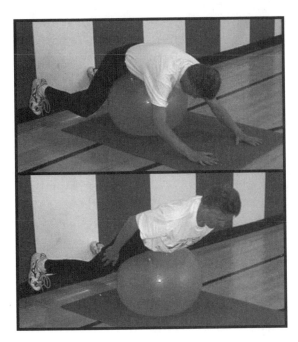

Upper Back Extension:

Lie belly down on top of the ball with your feet braced against a wall or other solid object. Your hands should be flat on the floor in front of the ball, approximately shoulder width apart. Tighten your abs and lift your upper torso off the ball, pushing with your feet to straighten your legs. Your body should be in a straight line. Do not arch your back. Hold 2–3 seconds, then slowly return to the starting position.

Lower Abdominal Crunch:

Lie on the floor, arms by your sides, palms down. Place the ball against your buttocks with both legs on top (as shown). Gripping the ball between your heels and your buttocks, lift both the ball and your buttocks off the floor. Slowly curl the lower part of your body toward your chest. Hold 2–3 seconds, then slowly lower the ball to the starting position.

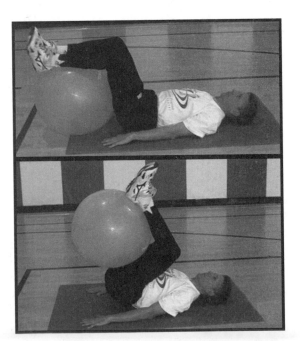

Double Leg Curl:

Lie on the floor with your arms by your sides, palms down. Place your heels and the lower part of your calves on top of the ball. Pushing your heels into the ball, tighten your abs, and lift your buttocks off the floor. Stabilize the ball, then roll it in toward your buttocks, keeping your knees together. Hold 2–3 seconds, then slowly roll the ball back to the starting position.

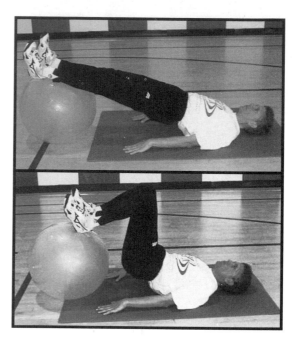

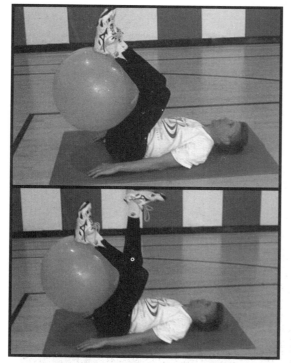

Hamstring Stretch:

Lie on the floor with your arms by your sides, palms down. Place the ball on the floor against your buttocks with your legs on top. Gripping the ball between your heels and buttocks, lift it off the floor. Holding the ball with one leg, extend the opposite leg (as shown). Lower your leg back to the ball and grab it with the heel and the buttocks. Extend the opposite leg. Continue alternating legs. One repetition includes both sides.

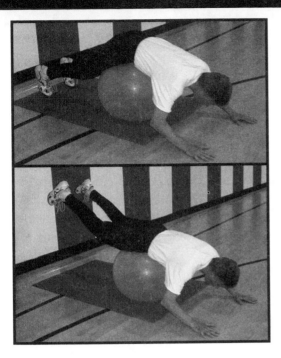

Lower Extension:

Lie on top of the ball as shown, hands flat on the floor with just your toes touching the floor. Lift your legs until your body is in a straight line. Do not arch your back. Hold 2–3 seconds, then slowly lower legs to the starting position.

Wall Squat:

Stand with the ball between your lower back and the wall. With your knees slightly bent, lean slightly into the ball. Grasp the medicine ball between your hands at the waist, elbows along your sides. If you do not have a medicine ball, clasp your hands together. Slowly roll the large ball down the wall until you are in a squatting position. As you squat, extend the medicine ball between your knees toward the floor. As you roll the ball back up to a standing position, extend the medicine ball in front of you, arms extended. Bring the medicine ball back to the starting position and repeat.

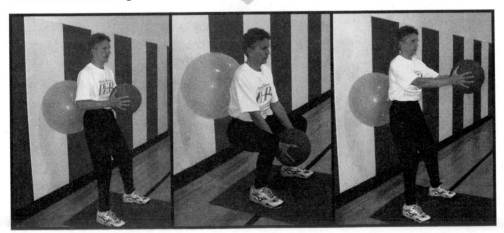

Rotation Program
Exercise Ball and Tubing

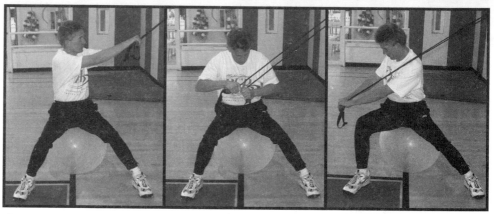

Chop:

Sit on the exercise ball with the tube anchored to a solid surface above shoulder height on one side. During this exercise, your eyes should follow your hands. Start with your arms extended far enough away from the tube for there to be tension. Holding the handles in both hands, pull them toward the chest. Pause. Turn to the opposite side and thrust the handles down to the side in a controlled motion. Return to a starting position in a controlled motion and repeat for the required reps. Repeat on the opposite side.

Lift:

Sit on the exercise ball with the tube anchored to a solid surface below shoulder height on one side. During this exercise, your eyes should follow your hands. Start with your arms extended far enough away from the tube for there to be tension. Holding the handles in both hands, pull them toward the chest. Pause. Turn away from the wall and thrust the handles up to the side in a controlled motion. Return to a starting position in a controlled motion and repeat for the required reps. Repeat on the opposite side.

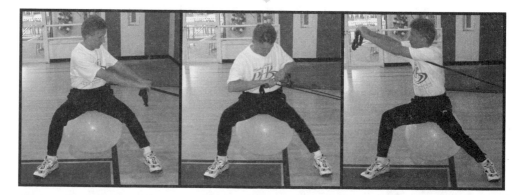

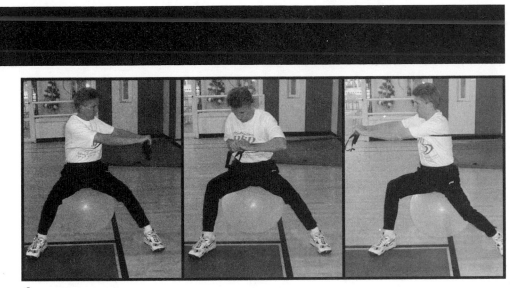

¹/₂ Rotation:

Sit on the exercise ball with the tube anchored to a solid surface parallel to shoulder height on one side. During this exercise, your eyes should follow your hands. Start with your arms extended far enough away from the tube for there to be tension. Holding the handles in both hands, pull them toward the chest. Pause. Turn away from the wall and thrust the handles out to the side in a controlled motion. Return to a starting position in a controlled motion and repeat for the required reps. Repeat on the opposite side.

Remember, work at your own pace and steadily increase the number of repetitions you perform. If you feel discomfort during any of the exercises, stop, reposition, and begin again. If your discomfort continues, consult a trainer at your gym regarding form or consult your physician if pain develops or discomfort persists.

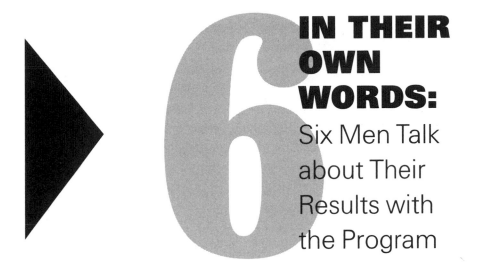

IN THEIR OWN WORDS:

Six Men Talk about Their Results with the Program

To me, the proof of the exercise and nutritional programs that I advocate are in the results. Whether I am working with world-class athletes who want to improve their already extraordinary performance or ordinary men who need to lose inches, gain strength, and build up their health profile, all the programs I design are based upon what I see happening in their bodies.

The six test subjects who followed my program to lose their love handles and build strength in the core area of their bodies had remarkable results in as little as 30 days. They lost inches in the waist area, lowered their BMIs, lost scale pounds, and even lowered their fat to lean-muscle ratios. Most important, they all felt good about themselves and what they had accomplished. Each man told me that he had more energy, better ability to manage daily stress, and that he felt much healthier. Friends, family members, and colleagues noticed the changes in their bodies and complimented the men on how good they were looking. One man told me that for years he had been embarrassed to take off his shirt because of abdominal fat, but that, after 2 months on the program, he felt good about taking off his shirt

119

because he had muscle definition again and could show off his chest and abdomen with pride.

I'm going to let the men tell you about how they benefited from the program in their own words. As I interviewed them, they didn't pull any punches and were very honest about their experiences with each aspect of the program.

I think every man reading this book may find a little bit of himself here and a great deal of positive motivation as he begins his own diet, aerobic walking, and resistance exercises. I begin each section with a progress chart so that you can see the remarkable results these men had achieved after 6 weeks, 10 weeks, and 14 weeks.

Bob is a 37-year-old police officer who is 6' ½" tall. Bob had exercised, run, and lifted weights off and on for the last 15 years, but found that he wasn't getting the results he wanted. "I'd been working pretty hard for the last few years, and I thought I'd gotten to a plateau that I wasn't going to get off till I left the earth." He was surprised and pleased at the results he was able to get in just 4 weeks and even happier with the results after 8 weeks. "I feel stronger. I'm happier looking in the mirror. I can notice the difference more in my stomach and where my oblique muscles are located. There's not as much fat there as there used to be."

The low-glycemic index diet was an important component of the program for Bob. He was more aware of the role of nutrition in training insulin than some of the other guys because he had suffered from hypoglycemia when he was 33 years old, and his doctor had given him a diet to control that condition. He saw certain differences between that food plan and mine, however. His doctor had told him to eat 5 or 6 times a day, but had warned him that almost all carbohydrates were "bad" for him. Bob told me that he didn't really follow that program like he should have. I suspect that part of his problem might have been that when a person tries to follow a low-carbohydrate diet, they feel tired and run-down all the time.

Bob admitted that his recent eating habits had not been all that they should be. He never ate breakfast, but ate an enormous lunch and supper. It was not unusual for him to eat supper at 11:00 at night, which meant, of course, that his body stored most of that food as fat while he slept. He did eat a wide variety of foods, however—fruits, vegetables, meat, and potatoes. And he loves pasta. But he was giving his metabolism the wrong message by feeding his body only twice a day.

Not being a breakfast person, Bob had a little difficulty getting into the habit of eating the prescribed breakfast, but he made sure that he always ate

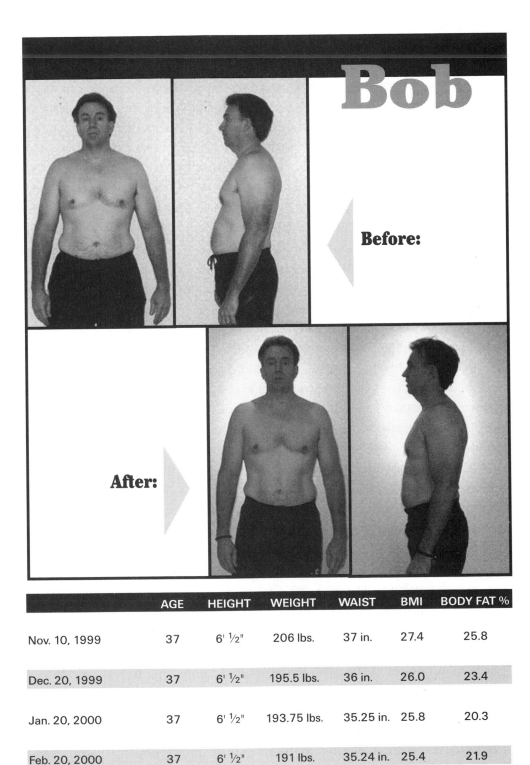

	AGE	HEIGHT	WEIGHT	WAIST	BMI	BODY FAT %
Nov. 10, 1999	37	6' ½"	206 lbs.	37 in.	27.4	25.8
Dec. 20, 1999	37	6' ½"	195.5 lbs.	36 in.	26.0	23.4
Jan. 20, 2000	37	6' ½"	193.75 lbs.	35.25 in.	25.8	20.3
Feb. 20, 2000	37	6' ½"	191 lbs.	35.24 in.	25.4	21.9

FIGURE 6.2 BOB'S MEASUREMENTS

something, even if it was just a glass of orange juice with Personal Edge Fat Metabolizer Protein Powder followed by a slice of toast. He really noticed the difference in energy that he got from eating five times per day. What pleased him the most was the fact that he was never hungry on my food plan—and he was surprised at how much food he could eat and still be within the parameters of the program. For most of the men, this was a pleasant change from the idea of "dieting," which implied being hungry and not feeling very energetic.

As for the aerobic part of the program, Bob did not feel that it was a hardship for him to fit in 45 minutes per day. Because of his work schedule and his obligations to the after-school activities of his daughter, he was not always able to do his walking before dinner. On those days, he made sure he walked in the morning before work rather than miss it. "I've found if you keep going, it's a lot harder to miss. If you miss a day here and a day there, it becomes a chore, a lot harder to get back into." Like most of the men, Bob felt that consistency was key to the program's overall success. He also mentioned that he had noticed that doing aerobic activity before dinner had a definite affect on his appetite. In fact, years ago when he used to jog, he had always noticed that he ate less.

What Bob really liked about the aerobic part of the program were the wide range of choices available to him. "You can choose what you want to do. You can ride a bike, walk, skip rope, and you don't have to push yourself. You don't have to beat yourself to death, to run a marathon every day that really tires you out."

Bob had no problem at all doing the core resistance exercises. They took him about 25 to 30 minutes a session, and he was able to work up to the prescribed number of sets pretty quickly and was faithful about doing them three to four times per week. He also continued with his circuit training routine at the gym. He told me that he really was happy to add my exercises to his routine, however, because he had never been able to get a really good abdominal workout, and he knew that having proper abdominal strength was important for keeping the lower back strong and pain free.

When I asked Bob if he found it difficult to follow this program during the holiday season, he admitted that it had been a little tough on Thanksgiving Day, which fell a week after the program began. But he went on to say, "To tell you the truth, I really felt better after I ate Thanksgiving dinner. In the afternoon, I'm usually sitting around. My stomach's out to there, and I can't move off the sofa. But this year, I really felt a difference. I didn't fill myself up as much."

When I asked Bob if he thought he would continue following the program, he replied, "I'm going to try and keep up with it because I'm happy with it, and I'm happy with the results."

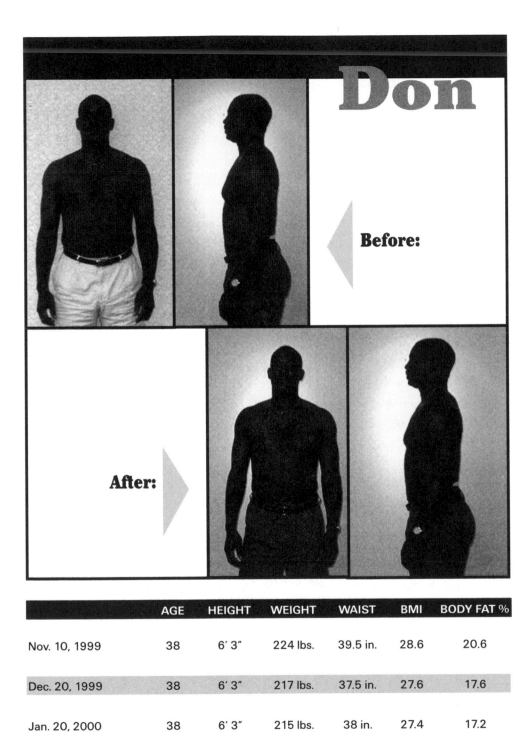

	AGE	HEIGHT	WEIGHT	WAIST	BMI	BODY FAT %
Nov. 10, 1999	38	6′ 3″	224 lbs.	39.5 in.	28.6	20.6
Dec. 20, 1999	38	6′ 3″	217 lbs.	37.5 in.	27.6	17.6
Jan. 20, 2000	38	6′ 3″	215 lbs.	38 in.	27.4	17.2
Feb. 20, 2000	38	6′ 3″	215 lbs.	37 in.	27.4	16

FIGURE 6.4 DON'S MEASUREMENTS

Don is 38 years old, 6' 3" tall, and teaches school for a living. He also coaches young boys' team sports after school many evenings, so he has a busy schedule, teaching from 7:00 to 5:00 during the day, and then coaching from 5:00 to 7:00 at night.

During his college years, Don was a defensive back on the Tulane University football team. When he graduated, he weighed 185 pounds and had 13.5 percent body fat. For 10 years, he had never got over 200 pounds, but in the last five he noticed that he was starting to put on body fat, especially in the abdominal area. At one point, his weight even got as high as 240. A big wake-up call for Don was the drop in his energy level. "I had always been energetic, and I had a high metabolic rate and a lot of endurance. I was able to go and do a lot of things and not get tired. But in the last five years, I felt physically drained. I was very tired and it was affecting my mental and emotional state in terms of concentrating. That's why I knew I had to get back into the gym and back to working out. I started playing baseketball for some conditioning and started doing some swimming, but I still felt deprived of energy. I couldn't maintain things that I wanted to do. I would be burnt at the end of a day, especially if I had a game after work and had a full basketball game or a football game."

From his background as an athlete, Don knew that there was a direct correlation between body weight and makeup, and physical activity. So he asked me if I could recommend a workout for him. I explained that I was looking for volunteers for a new program that, while not being geared toward an overall body workout, would tone the core area of the body. I also explained that the nutritional factor would help him to regain his lost energy. He was very interested and came to the orientation.

At the orientation, I gave the men a thorough grounding in the health risks associated with visceral abdominal fat. Don knew that men begin to put on fat as they approach the age of 40, but he had never understood what a risk factor it was for illnesses like type 2 diabetes and coronary problems, and that concerned him more than any other reason for losing abdominal fat. "I think the message got across to me and most of the guys who were there. We knew that body fat was a health risk, but we'd never heard about it the way that you actually put it." He immediately signed up for the program.

Don found the food plan to be different from his usual diet. "I usually ate a lot of all those glycemically unacceptable foods. I was a big bread eater, white bread and white starches, lots of rice, flour, biscuits, donuts, and different things like that. With your program, you made me more aware of what

I was eating, as opposed to how much—what's actually in the food, in the fruits, in the drinks. That way a person is able to at least moderate the things he eats. It's like a lifestyle management program." Don did admit that he couldn't give up the foods he'd eaten all his life overnight. At first he did some blending with the glycemically acceptable foods. Eventually, he was able to make a complete switch and feel good about it. One of the most important things that he realized was that a person might eat a large quantity of food, but that it was the *quality* of the food that gave you energy and strength. "Eating the types of food you had us on five times a day was beneficial in maintaining the strength and energy that I always had, which really helped me out."

Because of his busy schedule, Don found it difficult to avoid eating after 8:00 PM some evenings. "I did eat periodically after eight o'clock but usually I would have fruit, an apple, or some pears. Or drink some water and take some vitamins. And I didn't feel starved or hungry in the morning. When I got up, I'd follow the regimen: two egg whites, two bowls of Raisin Bran, an apple, some water, orange juice, and I'd take my vitamin supplements. My snack would always include an orange and an apple. And my lunch would be a cold-water fish, usually tuna fish salad with tomatoes. I'd use olive oil as a salad dressing.

"When I got that hunger craving, I ate Ritz Whole Wheat Crackers, about four or five, during the day, and I'd get some peanut butter and a fruit. I consistently had about two liters of water every day. A lot of frequent urination, for sure. But it was effective because it kept me balanced with my workload."

For Don, the whole key to sticking with the food plan was consistency, even when he slipped up for one meal. "I know some people go astray just out of habit. But if you stay close to it, stay consistent, you will not feel deprived or hungry or feel the need to eat late at night. And even if you do stray and eat a large meal, because of your consistency, you will be able to compensate because of the abdominal training you're doing. I had no idea how reducing body fat within the midsection area would stabilize the entire body."

For Don, the hardest part of the program was finding the time to get in his aerobic walking because his schedule required leaving early in the morning and getting home late at night. But he did the best he could with it and was sure to be especially faithful with the other two parts of the program.

Like most of the guys, Don had to work his way into the exercises. "I started off with fifteen reps. I know you said two sets of twenty-five, but I couldn't manage twenty-five because I had lost so much strength in my abdominal muscles. Then I moved up to two sets of twenty-five. Then I was able to do four sets of twenty-five. You just keep moving it up as your stomach gets stronger and stronger. As you gradually work yourself into it, then it will be more comfortable for you. In the beginning, I can't see anybody starting out doing two sets of twenty-five with the ball. It doesn't look like it's difficult, but the areas it works and the way it's designed take a lot of weight off your legs and put it directly onto your stomach, the target area in which you want to reduce body fat. That was effective because it did take a lot of weight off your legs. You couldn't use your legs or use your back. You were concentrating on using strictly the stomach muscles."

Don was very pleased with his results. "At night I used to feel worn out because my energy level would just be gone. But I feel revitalized and have a lot of energy since I've been on this program." Also he told me, "I was just amazed because I didn't know where I would be in terms of the numbers. I didn't have the time to work with a personal trainer, so I did it on my own." Although some of the guys in the program checked in with the trainers I made available to them to monitor their progress, I was glad to hear this because I had designed the program as something any reader could do at home and get good results without outside input.

Don also felt that the program was easy to make a part of his life. "It doesn't cost you a whole lot to do it, and it doesn't take a lot of time out of your schedule, nor is it strenuous. There are some programs that take strenuous exercise to reach a particular result. But I think exercise, rest, and foods that can give you the proper nutrients can be effective. Nothing else I've ever done works on your abdomen. Even with running, you're doing your legs, butt, back, hamstrings, and quads. Nothing else concentrates directly on that area. Once you get used to it, your body can get adjusted, and it becomes a part of you to the point where it's nothing strenuous; it's just natural."

As a teacher and coach, it is second nature to Don to share new ideas that work for him. He has become so enthusiastic about the program that he has passed it on to a couple of his college friends, who have experienced weight gains up to 280 pounds since they graduated. He even bought his wife a Swiss ball so that she could work out with him. Don is most excited about incorporating the program into the health classes that he teaches to the 5th through 8th grades. "I'll get the little balls and start teaching what this has given me to the kids at the early ages, like 2nd, 3rd, 4th, and 5th grades. And then in health class, with the nutrition, I can tell them about the glycemically acceptable and unacceptable foods. Can you imagine presenting that to 7th graders!" Actually, the thought makes me very happy.

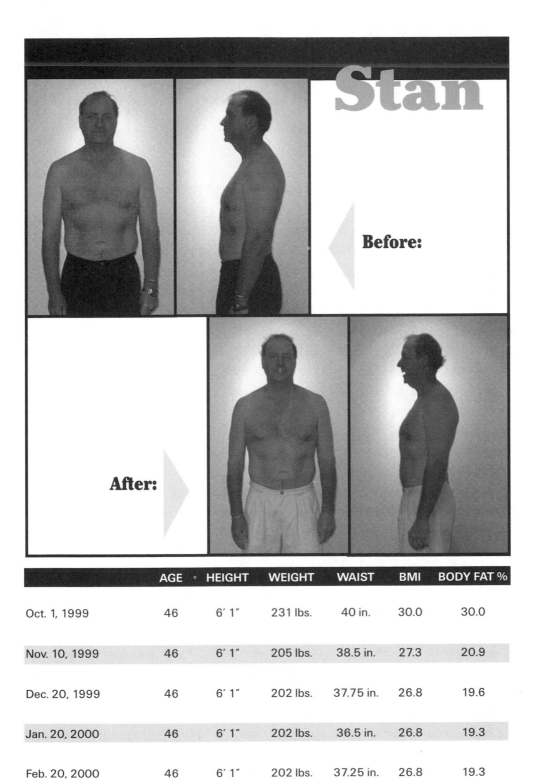

Stan

Before:

After:

	AGE	°	HEIGHT	WEIGHT	WAIST	BMI	BODY FAT %
Oct. 1, 1999	46		6′ 1″	231 lbs.	40 in.	30.0	30.0
Nov. 10, 1999	46		6′ 1″	205 lbs.	38.5 in.	27.3	20.9
Dec. 20, 1999	46		6′ 1″	202 lbs.	37.75 in.	26.8	19.6
Jan. 20, 2000	46		6′ 1″	202 lbs.	36.5 in.	26.8	19.3
Feb. 20, 2000	46		6′ 1″	202 lbs.	37.25 in.	26.8	19.3

FIGURE 6.6 STAN'S MEASUREMENTS

Stan is a 46-year-old golf pro who stands 6' 1" tall. Stan began the program about 6 weeks earlier than the other participants, so his losses are actually much greater. Stan began at 231 pounds. By the end of his first 6 weeks, he was down to 205 pounds, a loss of 26 pounds. By that time he had tightened his belt two notches and lowered his overall body fat from 30 percent to 20.9 percent.

Stan had been gaining weight for a number of years, but finally realized that he had to put a stop to it because it was hurting his game. "No matter what anyone says, golf is a strenuous sport to play professionally. To ride a cart around is one thing, but if you're going to be out there walking, and you have to compete with other people, you've got to practice two–three hours a day and play nonstop. It takes a lot out of you. If you're not in shape, you won't be able to give it the best effort of practice to *get* better. So, that's really part of the reason I wanted to get with this program." Stan's dream is to not only get in shape to become a better golfer, but to play the Senior Tour. Needless to say, he is *serious* about staying in the game.

Stan was the only person in the study who said that he felt hungry on the food plan. But he also admitted that not only had he been eating all the wrong things before, but in huge quantities. "I was consuming a tremendous amount of calories at each meal. I did a lot of work on that. It's a big difference with me because I used to eat weird stuff for breakfast, like pizza. For lunch, I ate five pieces of Popeye's fried chicken, which has about 500 calories per piece. I used to be so out of whack, and now I'm trying to watch all that stuff. I haven't had a piece of fried chicken since we started. Pizza, fried foods, beer, candy, sugar, potato chips, all those things that used to be my daily diet are gone now. It's tough to change overnight. It takes awhile, but I'm still doing it."

Stan felt that the exercise component of the program was vitally important. He had tried the Sugar Busters diet awhile back and managed to lose some weight on it, but he felt that, ultimately, his whole purpose had been defeated because he didn't exercise while he reduced. In the end, he gained back most of the weight. "If you don't exercise, you defeat the purpose of the diet. I wouldn't have gotten to where I am now if it hadn't been for the exercises. I think it's got to be a combination of all of the above."

Doing the exercises was hard for Stan in the beginning. "Because my waist and that whole area were so out of shape, they were really tough for me to do. As I've gone along, they've gotten a lot better. I still definitely have a ways to go, which is good, because I want a challenge." Stan combines my resistance exercises with specific exercises for golf, for a total workout time of 1½ to 2 hours per session. He has found that the two types of workouts complement each other beautifully—and have definitely improved his game.

One of the things Stan appreciates about combining the aerobic walking with the exercise program is that it takes the edge off his appetite. He does his walking at the end of his workday, before dinner, as recommended. Finding a place to walk was no problem for him. "I work at a golf course with a track around it, so I've got the availability to walk around the track at any time of the day. I can do it at night, I can do it on the treadmill at the health club, and I have a treadmill at home. All these things were available three months ago, and I didn't use them. Now I'm using them. So, that's a change." Stan found walking to be the most enjoyable part of the program. "I'd walk for forty-five to sixty minutes at a high pace and I'd definitely burn calories. Plus, when you're exercising a lot too, you've got a lot of things going for you."

When I asked Stan how he felt after doing the program for a couple of months, he said, "From my waist up, I feel a whole lot lighter. I guess that's probably, for the most part, where I have lost all the weight. My chest, and my arms and everything, feel a lot lighter. I think I'm a lot calmer. I haven't been tested, but I would say that my blood pressure and my pulse and everything are better. Obviously, that's not surprising if you lose twenty-six pounds. Obviously, when I had thirty percent body fat, that was ridiculous. When you get down to twenty percent when you're forty-seven years old, it's not that bad. But I want to try and get it down better. The more I can do, the more I know other people can do. You've just got to do it and to stick with it and be religious about it. It's got to be part of your daily routine. If you want to get yourself in better shape and get feeling better, you've got to put out."

When I asked Stan why he thought this program had worked so well for him, he said, "I guess everybody has done similar things, a little bit here and a little bit there. But, Mackie, you've just been doing this for so long, and you've got the athletes in your corner because you've trained athletes before. I think that's what gives this program a lot of credibility. I know that the people you've worked with are some of the biggest athletes, especially in boxing. You really have to be in shape if you've dealt with those kinds of people. That's your expertise. Certainly, if you can get those kinds of people in such tremendous shape, you can get the average guy to lose a little bit around his stomach. I'm really excited about it. Just talking to you now is going to make me try to stick to it a little bit more."

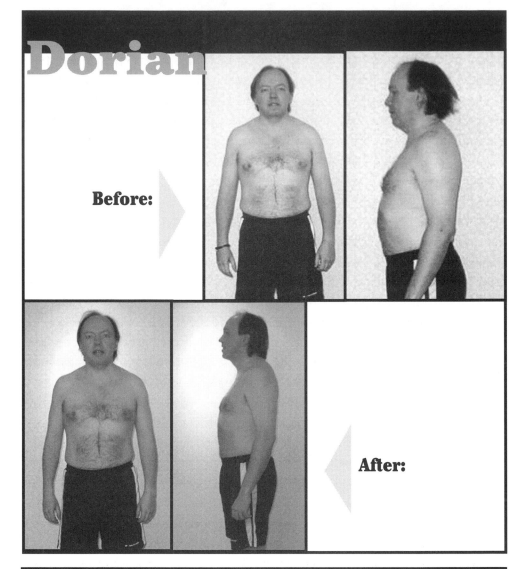

Dorian

Before:

After:

	AGE	HEIGHT	WEIGHT	WAIST	BMI	BODY FAT %
Nov. 10, 1999	46	5'10"	194 lbs.	38.5 in.	27.6	24.7
Dec. 20, 1999	46	5' 10"	187 lbs.	37 in.	26.6	23.5
Jan. 20, 2000	46	5' 10"	189 lbs.	37 in.	26.8	20.7
Feb. 20, 2000	46	5' 10"	188 lbs.	36 in.	26.7	21.3

FIGURE 6.8 DORIAN'S MEASUREMENTS

A professional real estate broker, Dorian is 46 years old and 5' 10" in height. He combines my program with his regular workout at the gym 3 days a week. Dorian's motivation for participating in this program was quality of life and building strength. A devoted father and family man, Dorian shared one of the most important reasons in his life for staying in shape. "I think this all came up for me a couple of years ago when my little girl was six years old. When she'd fall asleep, I'd carry her up to bed. It was getting to where I couldn't carry her up the stairs. She was just too heavy. I didn't want to give up on that. That's probably one of the big things. Now she's eight and I can carry her, no problem."

Dorian had tried to lose weight a few times in the past, but when I asked him if he had been successful in taking it off and keeping it off, he said, "Not really, not to any degree. And I've never really prescribed to any sort of programs. I resisted letting Jenny Craig or any of that stuff come into the house. And I had never really been involved in any serious exercise or fitness programs. I've always been somebody who was kind of stop and start."

Like many of the men who participated in the study, Dorian soon realized that following a good food plan was not just a common-sense proposition. Most of us don't know much about nutrition and need to learn more about it. "I was at a loss as to where to begin with all this stuff. If you don't know much about food, and I'm not one, you can talk about carbohydrates, and you can talk about proteins and different types of things. And I can maybe name a couple of things in whatever category. But I'm not really into it." Fortunately, Dorian was also able to rely on input from his wife, who is a superb cook, to plan low-glycemic meals for him and the rest of the family.

Like many people who live in New Orleans and can take advantage of one of our country's greatest regional cuisines, Dorian normally ate a lot of dishes that contained rice, a high-glycemic food. He also ate a lot of meat, potatoes, fish, pasta, and desserts. Sugar was hard for him to give up. "That's the biggest thing on the list. All those sugars have to go. And that's hard." But he did feel satisfied with the quantity of food he got to eat on the food plan. And he especially enjoyed having the Personal Edge Fat Metabolizer Protein shake and the low-glycemic protein bars as snacks. "You can mix the soy powder with apple juice and different types of things. That's very filling. And then those protein bars are pretty swell, too. You develop a taste for those. And I like the fiber stuff that my wife found for breakfast. I'm allergic to milk, so I've already been using rice milk and soy milk and all that, so that's an easy one for me."

When I asked Dorian if he had any difficulty doing the exercises, he said, "They were hard to begin with. It's a whole new set of muscles that you are working. And then you get to where you can handle the exercises and deal with them, but none of it was what you would call easy. You feel it, you really feel it. But I imagine that's what they're geared for. I always think that the exercises are called "dead bugs" because they're for all those parts of your body that never get worked out." (In exercise parlance, exercise programs are humorously called dead bugs because of the black and white pictures of men lying on their backs demonstrating the routines.) Dorian stressed that initially feeling the effort in his abdominal muscles was a very good thing. Like the other guys who had done some circuit training prior to the program, he felt that none of those machines had even really worked his abdominal area in the same way.

Dorian regarded his aerobic workout and the exercise program as enjoyable downtime from his stressful and busy day, a time when he could just turn off the phones and get away from it all. "It's relaxing for me to just not do anything but that for an hour and a half, two hours. It's a selfish kind of thing."

Dorian found that what worked best for his schedule was to do both his workout and his aerobic walking program in the early part of the day. "I'm a morning person. It's got to happen for me in the morning, or it just isn't going to happen. Basically, I drop my little girl off at school and I go over to the gym, and then I show up at work at 9:30 or 10:00. Of course, I've got that kind of flexibility because I own the place. But I imagine you can create that kind of flexibility, no matter where you work, just as long as you set it up. If you do a good job, nobody really cares when you do it, as long as you do it. At least that's the way I think." Dorian was also very faithful about doing the aerobic walking at least five times a week and doing the exercises the prescribed three or four times. In fact, he would sometimes do them more often, which is a plus with abdominal exercises because that part of the body is actually designed to take frequent workouts. All the more reason why we "go to pot" when we don't work those muscles.

When I asked Dorian whether it was hard for him to stick with the program around the holidays, he laughed, saying he suspected that was a little joke on my part, suggesting that the guys follow this program during that time of year. But he managed to stick with it, even though he felt a bit deprived on Thanksgiving Day.

Dorian told me that he intends to stick with the program. He likes the way he feels and everyone he knows is giving him plenty of positive feedback on the changes in his appearance. And that makes him feel great.

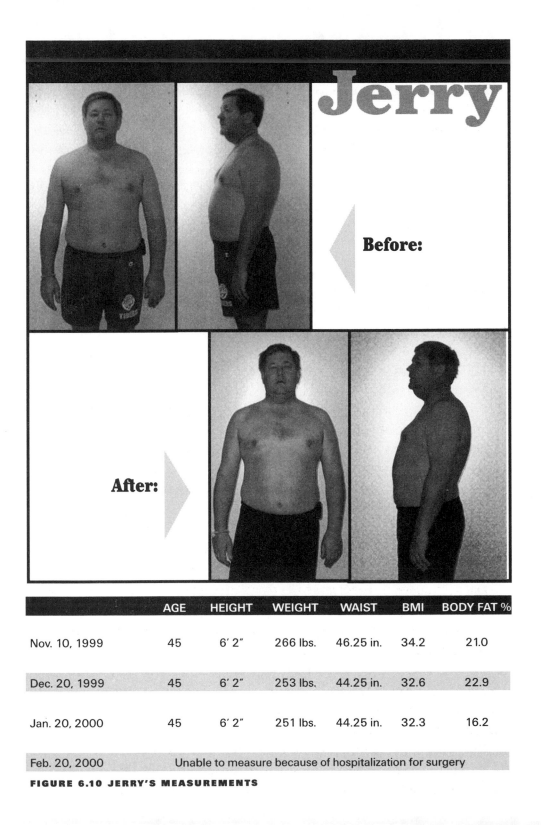

	AGE	HEIGHT	WEIGHT	WAIST	BMI	BODY FAT %
Nov. 10, 1999	45	6′ 2″	266 lbs.	46.25 in.	34.2	21.0
Dec. 20, 1999	45	6′ 2″	253 lbs.	44.25 in.	32.6	22.9
Jan. 20, 2000	45	6′ 2″	251 lbs.	44.25 in.	32.3	16.2
Feb. 20, 2000	Unable to measure because of hospitalization for surgery					

FIGURE 6.10 JERRY'S MEASUREMENTS

Jerry is a 45-year-old police officer. We were not able to get his statistics for the dates between January 20 and February 20th because he was hospitalized for three weeks due to major abdominal surgery. This surgery was organic in nature—in other words, he did not injure himself while doing the program. Within a month of his being released from the hospital, however, he was back in the gym recovering the ground that he had lost. As of this writing, he's still with the program and doing great.

Jerry told me that he signed up for the program "because of the confidence I have in you." But another big motivation for him was going to the orientation and hearing about the health risks associated with abdominal fat. "It opened up my eyes. I'll say that. I was taken aback by some of the stuff you were saying. I don't think the average person has any idea. Afterward, talking to the other guys in the study, that was a big topic of conversation. The average guy was just shocked."

Jerry had tried some diet and exercise regimens over the years, but he was discouraged by the amount of time these programs took up and the food limitations of the diets. "A lot of diets I've tried over the years, you live hungry."

One of the things that Jerry most appreciated about my 30-day program was the quality of the low-glycemic food plan. "I was never hungry. There were two snacks and then three meals a day. I probably ate more on this than on any other diet, and I probably ate right." He admitted that my food plan was more restrictive in some respects than his normal diet. "But it wasn't a problem. I don't have a problem with seafood, the fish and the salmon. The only complaint I had about the diet was that I found that it was difficult at lunchtime on a workday, or eating out—to find the salmon or to get them to cook the chicken the right way. I didn't find that easy. At home, it's a piece of cake."

Jerry's wife became so enthusiastic about the food plan and the meals she could cook with it that the whole family is now eating low-glycemic foods. "I have twin boys and two girls, and I think that we all are eating healthier because of my diet." Jerry also commented that he liked the soy drink I recommended for snacks. "Some of that stuff can be wicked tasting, and I didn't find that the case at all with the soy."

Jerry did most of his aerobic walking in the morning, but did manage to do some of it in the late afternoon or evening. Since his work is so demanding, he found that he could use his walking time to be with his family. "Many times the wife would join me. The boys would come out on their bikes and ride along, so it was a good thing. I thought that was one of the pluses. And if you're walking in the neighborhood, as opposed to the treadmill, forty-five minutes just shoots by."

When I asked Jerry if he had any problems initially doing the exercises, he said he had been able to ease into them pretty well. "Within a week I was able to do them without any problem. It did take me about a week to work up to forty-five minutes of walking. Twenty-five minutes or thirty-five was not a problem, but the last ten minutes was hard for me at first."

One of the things Jerry liked most about the program was how the time frame fit so well into his busy life. "I'm a police captain. I put in a lot of hours, that's just the nature of the beast. And then you're on call. Here in New Orleans, you can imagine we get a lot of special events. A lot of that comes under my umbrella. So you run and go all the time. And if you want to spend any time at all at home with the family, it's even more of a problem. That's what I thought was really good about the program, the exercise did not eat up your day. You could easily fit it into the morning. I'd say 60 to 70 percent of the time I went to the gym in the morning, before the workday started. But if I had early morning meetings or whatever, it was easy to fit into the afternoons."

Jerry also said that he had a lot more energy now. "I do have more energy, without question. I feel healthy, better about myself. Over the two months, I lost around thirteen pounds and almost three inches. I could really feel a difference in the waistline of my pants. Of course, the comments you get from family and friends, obviously that helps out too."

Jerry liked the program so much that he said he was going to make it "a permanent fixture in my life." He also planned to mix it with some resistance exercises at the gym, a practice I always recommend if you want to see more overall results in the rest of your body.

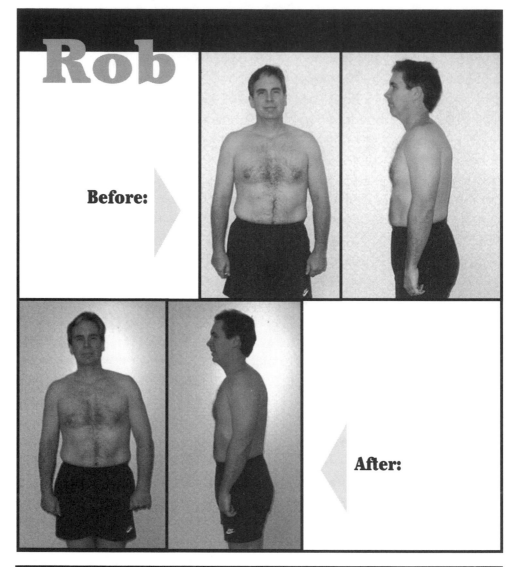

Rob

Before:

After:

	AGE	HEIGHT	WEIGHT	WAIST	BMI	BODY FAT %
Nov. 10, 1999	44	5' 11"	197.5 lbs.	39.25 in.	27.7	22.9
Dec. 20, 1999	44	5' 11"	193 lbs.	38 in.	27.1	19.1
Jan. 20, 2000	44	5' 11"	194 lbs.	37 in.	27.2	21.5
Feb. 20, 2000	44	5' 11"	193 lbs.	37.5 in.	27.1	19.1

FIGURE 6.12 ROB'S MEASUREMENTS

Rob is a 44-year-old police officer who stands 5' 11". In the past, Rob had participated off and on in some of the programs that I had designed. When he heard some of the guys talking enthusiastically about this one, he asked me about it, and I invited him to sign up.

Rob had also tried the Sugar Busters diet before and had lost 28 pounds on it. He said he was able to keep the weight off "somewhat." What had helped him in that area was joining a gym and working out regularly. I wasn't surprised to hear him say that because I know diet and exercise are always the magic combination if you want to lose fat.

Because of the kind of food plan he had been on before, Rob was no stranger to the glycemic index, but he did notice some differences between my plan and Sugar Busters, especially in the area of incorporating more carbohydrates into the diet. Rob had only been eating three meals a day and added in the two snacks that I suggested. He was also surprised to see himself losing inches before he lost scale weight. That was not surprising to me, however, because, as I said earlier, scale weight is a very unreliable indicator of positive changes in the body.

Basically, Rob found the food plan very easy to follow. "If you can't modify the way you eat using these acceptable foods, then I don't see how you could do it at all. This is really simple. You can go into a restaurant and pick and choose what to eat and still stay on track."

Since Rob has a second job and must fit his workout into the hour and 10 minute period between one job and the next, he had a bit of trouble doing the minimum 45 minutes of aerobic walking. But he tried to do what he could. "Some days I might be able to do it for 15 minutes, or it may be 20 or 25. But I still got on the treadmill and did it." He also added that the hour and 10 minutes it takes him to work out was "hardly any time at all on the grand scale of things when you really think about it."

Rob combined the exercises I prescribed for the program with some circuit training he was already doing. In fact, he said that he "fell right into" some of the exercises. He was able to get through the two sets on the Swiss ball in about 10 minutes. At first, however, he was concerned that he might feel some strain because the core area of his body was somewhat weak. "I was worried about that because of the way I felt directly after the exercises. But in the long run they actually made me feel better, especially my lower back. It was tough the first few times. I'm not going to lie. For me, it was actually a little painful. But after I dressed and got into the car, I didn't feel any aftereffects after the first couple of times. And now it's nothing. I know it's working. I really like it."

When I asked Rob whether he found it hard to keep doing the exercises three to four times a week, I got a big kick out of his answer. "It's missing the workout routine that's difficult. It's more difficult to miss it than to do it. I feel worse when I don't go. Like this Wednesday, I won't be able to make it, and I'm dreading that." I laughed and told him that I'd never heard anyone say that they dreaded *missing* exercise. Usually they dread *doing* it. Rob added that the workout made him feel great. "No doubt about it. The way I feel when I leave there is just hard to describe."

As of this writing, the six men who spent 2 months following my food, aerobic walking, and exercise plans are all continuing to follow my program because it's easy for them to keep getting these great results without taking too big a time chunk out of their daily lives. I figure that if they can get such fantastic results during the biggest and most stressful holiday season of the year, Thanksgiving, and Christmas and Hanukkah, no reader has any real excuse not to give this program a try. If you want to lose inches in your waistline, improve your health and longevity, radically decrease your vulnerability to serious diseases such as type 2 diabetes and heart disease, and feel and look like a new man, this is the program for you. So, what are you waiting for? Both literally and figuratively, it's the chance of a lifetime.

7 FREQUENTLY ASKED QUESTIONS

Whenever I talk about exercise, managing insulin, and losing weight in the abdominal area, I find that people frequently ask me specific questions. One of the reasons for this is that there is so much misinformation about weight loss, how to achieve good health through lifestyle modification, and what constitutes good nutrition. To clarify some of the most important points that I have discussed in this book, I am including a special review chapter of common questions and answers.

Question: Is scale weight the most reliable indication of whether or not a person is in good health?

Answer: Many people in this culture constantly weigh themselves to see how "thin" they are. While scale weight certainly has something to do with our health and general well-being, it is less important than body composition, the ratio of fat to lean-muscle that we carry. A nutritionist friend of mine has two plastic representations in his office: 5 pounds of lean muscle looks like a couple of filet mignons piled on top of one another; 5 pounds of fat is about four times larger and looks like a huge glob of yellow fluff.

Obviously, you would rather have the 5 pounds of lean muscle inside of your body than the unappealing 5-pound glob of fat.

Weight according to the scale tells us little about the really important health factors, such as our ability to manage insulin and the efficiency of our metabolism. Two men of similar height can have identical weights, 165 pounds. But if one man is lean and toned and the other is out of condition, scale weight will not be a reliable indication of which man is in good health. Conversely, a man who is 20 to 30 pounds overweight, but exercises regularly and eats a nutritionally balanced, low-glycemic food plan will be less at risk for heart disease, type 2 diabetes, and hypertension than a man who is close to the "scale weight" for his height, but does not exercise or eat nutritionally. Again, the key is body composition.

Question: If I had to choose one body measurement to indicate my health risks, would I choose my body fat percentage or my waist measurement?

Answer: The circumference of the waist is, without a doubt, the most important and reliable indicator of health risks. According to the *Canadian Journal of Diabetes Care,* an increase in the waist is always a clear indicator that excess fat is collecting in the abdominal area, especially in men between the ages of 40 and 60 years. In one 7-year study, even though the subjects' scale weight and BMI remained the same, there was a marked increase in the waist measurement accompanied by a 30 percent increase in abdominal fat. The subjects also became more insulin resistant over this time period, becoming prime candidates for type 2 diabetes. When a man's waist circumference exceeds 40 inches, he is not only at greater risk for developing type 2 diabetes, but also higher cholesterol levels, which often leads to coronary disease.

An increasing waistline signifies what I call "creeping obesity." If you know your waist measurement is steadily increasing, even if your weight in pounds is not, now is the time to take steps to bring that measurement down. If a man's waist has reached 40 inches by the time he is 40 years old, he's in big trouble because the problem will only get worse as he moves into his 50's, 60's, and 70's (if he lives that long).

Question: Is it just aging that causes fat gain? What other factors contribute?

Answer: Absolutely not. A man can have a healthy body fat to lean-muscle ratio and an efficient metabolism at any age if he is willing to keep his body fit. We are born with fat cells in our body, but we are not born fat. What causes us to gain fat, especially in the abdominal area, is overeating, poor nutrition, a sedentary lifestyle, and lack of exercise. The typical American high-fat, high-sugar diet, which is based on processed and fast foods, makes us insulin resistant, leading to greater storage of food energy in the fat cells. Take a 20-year-old man who is 5' 10" tall, weighs 160 pounds, and has only 15 percent fat in his body composition; a healthy amount of body fat for the average man. By the time this man reaches the age of 40, he may now weigh 185 pounds and have 25 percent body fat. This is not because he is getting older, but because his more demanding work schedule and lifestyle have caused him to gradually become less physically active and to eat more fast foods. He might be so busy that he skips meals on a regular basis, causing his metabolism to become less efficient at burning calories since his body thinks that there is a famine going on. And he probably gets less sleep than he did as a young man due to the heavy responsibilities of career and family. Add to this the fat-storing properties of the constant stress he is under. And because fat burns fewer calories than muscle, he is setting himself up for still more weight gain, greater insulin resistance, and possibly some serious health risks in later life due to a slower metabolism (less lean muscle to burn calories). Aging alone does not cause us to gain a greater percentage of body fat. Our decreasing level of activity and the foods that we eat as we grow older are the primary culprits.

Question: Will someone in his 30's derive greater benefit from this program than someone in his 40's, 50's, 60's, or even 70's?

Answer: Over the past 25 years as a performance enhancement consultant to athletes who wished to extend their careers past normal retirement age, and to thousands of ordinary men and women, I have seen that age is no barrier to becoming physically fit and healthy. Our bodies have evolved to work hard and efficiently. That's nature's design—and she's had a million years to perfect it.

I recently received a wonderful letter from John "Rocky" Roe, a Major League Baseball umpire. Rocky came to me at my Center for Performance Enhancement and Lifestyle Management at the age of 49 to see if my program could help him. Over a period of just 2 months, Rocky achieved incredible losses in pounds and inches across the board. I have included his statistics below:

Date:	Age:	Height	Weight	Waist	BMI	Body Fat %
Feb.29	49	6′	312	57.5″	42.34	39
April.24	49	6′	278	52.5″	40	35

FIGURE 7.1: STATISTICS FOR JOHN "ROCKY" ROE, FEBRUARY 2000 TO APRIL 2000

When I asked him to write about his experience for this book, here is what he sent to me:

> Mackie Shilstone's program really saved my life (literally). I came to Mackie to try to change my lifestyle. I committed to the program wholeheartedly, and I lost a total of 34 pounds over a 2½-month period. A by-product of his testing found me to have high blood sugar, high cholesterol, and some potential heart problems. Through Mackie's persistence, he provided me with the clinical help that will allow me to live a long and prosperous life. I did have a knee injury, and Mackie provided me with state-of-the-art physical therapy. Lastly, he provided me with an aftercare program that has made my knee healthy again. Thanks to Mackie, not only is the rehab of my knee going great, but also he has truly touched my life and changed it for the better.

Letters such as this make me feel as if all my work is worthwhile and, over the years I have received many similar written and verbal endorsements and thanks for my program. No matter what your age, I can guarantee that if you consistently follow the program described in this book, you will experience a decrease in your waistline and BMI, greater energy levels, abdominal fat loss, and a more toned and fit core area of the body.

Question: Can this program help me to lower my total cholesterol if it is too high?
Answer: Yes. Scientific research has shown conclusively that regular exercise and proper nutrition not only lower one's overall cholesterol level, but can also increase one's percentage of HDL (good cholesterol) vs. LDL (bad cholesterol).

Question: If I don't exercise, but just eat the food plan recommended in this book, will I still lose weight?

Answer: There is no doubt that matching your daily caloric intake to your body type and consistently eating low-glycemic foods in the proper proportions of 55 percent carbohydrates, 20 percent lean protein, and 25 percent acceptable fat, will cause you to lose weight. In fact, you can lose pounds by following almost any of the popular diets out there. But studies have shown that people usually gain back a significant amount of the weight lost within the first 6 months of going off the diet plan. If you want to keep your weight off and maintain a health body composition (fat to lean-muscle ratio), you need to add exercise to your program. Current research shows that making regular exercise and cardio-training a part of your life not only helps you to take off weight faster by increasing your metabolism (your ability to burn fat), it is the only way that has been clinically proven to keep weight off in the long run. As we age, resistance exercises and proper nutrition become key to maintaining our health and longevity. This combination also increases the amount of pounds lost from fat and minimizes loss of lean muscle mass.

The American College of Sports Medicine states that exercise is one of the most effective ways of controlling insulin resistance. When our insulin response is normalized, our bodies will be able to more efficiently use the fuel we put into it and store less as fat.

Question: Why does eating complex (low-glycemic) foods lead to a stable insulin response?

Answer: Complex foods, which include things such as whole grains, legumes, and vegetables that have a high fiber content, are low in simple sugars and take longer to digest. The glycemic index rates foods according to the speed at which they are digested and converted to energy or stored as fat. Low-glycemic foods are more complex and require burning more calories to digest them. High-glycemic foods digest quickly. If they are not burned during daily activities, they are usually stored as fat because the body is programmed to store the food energy that we cannot use immediately.

Carbohydrates stimulate the secretion of insulin more than any other type of food. When we eat low-glycemic (complex) carbohydrates, such as whole wheat bread, oatmeal, and yams, the pancreas doesn't have to work as hard because these carbohydrates take time to digest. Therefore, more of them get burned as energy rather than stored in the fat cells when a diet

143

consists mainly of simple carbohydrates, such as white bread, sugary breakfast cereals, fast foods, and high-calorie desserts—foods that are easily and quickly converted into glucose—the pancreas can become over-stimulated. If the latter type of eating pattern goes on over a long period of time, the pancreas becomes "exhausted," leading to conditions such as type 1 or type 2 diabetes, hypertension, heart disease, and high cholesterol.

Consistently eating low-glycemic foods that digest at a slower rate, especially complex carbohydrates, normalizes the insulin response and decreases the amount of glucose our body must store as fat because it has no immediate use for it.

Question: Will eating this low-glycemic food plan increase my energy level?
Answer: Eating this food plan will not only increase your energy level, it will also stabilize your energy level. When people skip meals or do not space them evenly throughout the day, their insulin levels yo-yo up and down, causing them to have energy highs and lows.

Question: Will I be harming myself if I occasionally eat a high-glycemic food?
Answer: No. It is not just *what* we eat that creates a stabile insulin response, but what foods *with which* we eat something. If, for example, you eat a high-glycemic banana with some low-glycemic protein, the 2 foods will even out to give you a moderate glycemic response on average. Typically, athletes will tend to eat more low-glycemic foods the closer they get to a competitive event. Right after the event, they will eat high-glycemic foods, progressing to moderate-glycemic foods, to help them to recover and bring their energy levels back up. This is especially important if one is participating in multiple events.

Question: What if I allow the low glycemic carbohydrates in my diet to go under the recommended 55 percent?
Answer: The carbohydrates that we eat provide our body with needed energy. To maintain the brain and central nervous system, the body needs a certain amount of glucose, which it gets from sugars and starches, the by-products of carbohydrates after digestion. The body stores this glucose in the liver and in the muscles. Some of the popular diets out there suggest that you keep your carbohydrate intake low. This may cause weight loss in the short run, but it will also create low energy levels because your body will not have enough of this high-energy food source. You could also lose

lean muscle weight if the percentage of carbohydrates in your diet goes too low and your stress levels go up.

If you are not eating enough carbs, the body has to get its supply from somewhere, so it will begin breaking down muscle protein to synthesize glucose to supply your vital organs with an adequate supply. The weight you lose will be muscle, not fat, because your body cannot break down its fat stores into glycogen. The goal of a good weight loss program should always be to lose as little muscle as possible in comparison to fat loss. If you exercise while on a low carbohydrate diet, that will make you more prone to lose lean muscle instead of fat.

Question: What if I eat more than 60 percent low glycemic carbohydrates?
Answer: The result you want is to eat enough carbohydrates to provide your body with sufficient fuel, but not so many that it begins to store them as fat. In my experience, and according to many researchers and nutritionists, 55 percent is the ideal amount of carbohydrates to ingest.

Question: Will I lose weight more quickly and be healthier if I only buy foods whose labels say "low-fat"?
Answer: Never before have their been so many foods labeled "low-fat" or "fat-free" on the market—and never before have Americans been so fat. Dr. Ann de Wees Allen of the Glycemic Institute warns that such labeling can be highly deceiving. When the fats are taken out of foods, manufacturers most often replace them with sugars and carbohydrates to make up for the lost flavor. But, ironically, the fats that have been removed from these foods were not as fattening as the sugars that have replaced them.

I recommend that people stay away from processed fat-free foods. Instead, stick with low-glycemic foods where you know what you are getting and never have to worry about any hidden, high-caloric ingredients and flavor enhancers.

Question: How do I know if the foods I am buying in the supermarket are flavored with sugars that are low-glycemic?
Answer: Not all sugars are created equal. "Bad" sugars include maltodextrins, glucose and glucose polymers, invert sugar, dextrose, raw sugars, honey, brown sugar, barley malt, date sugar, turbinado sugar, cane sugar, maple sugar, carmelized sugar, and blackstrap molasses. All of these sugars are high-glycemic and elevate blood sugar, making you more insulin resist-

ant. While sucrose has a lower glycemic index than these other sugars, studies have shown that it has long-term negative health effects and has actually been shown to increase the risk of heart disease in the 20 percent of the population who have elevated serum triglyceride levels.

Read the labels on the processed foods and low-fat desserts before you buy them. You may find that you have been filling your kitchen with "diet" foods that cause you to actually *gain* weight, rather than *lose* it. Research has also shown that high-glycemic sugars also work to suppress the immune system. Cancer cells thrive on them.

Your best choices are foods sweetened with fruit sugars made from low-glycemic fruits. The type of fruit sugar in a product will always be listed on the label.

Question: Why should I eat my fruits separately?

Answer: Harvey Diamond, author of *Fit for Life—A New Beginning: Your Complete Diet and Health Plan for the Millennium,* and who was recently a guest on my radio show, makes the point that fruit takes about 45 minutes to digest in the small intestine. If there is something ahead of it, it gets held in the intestinal track longer and does not completely digest, causing putrefaction, discomfort, and gas. When we eat fruits with sugary desserts, the fruit has a tendency to convert to alcohol in the digestive track. When glycemically acceptable fruits are eaten between meals, they become a stabilizing factor because they help to normalize the insulin response by keeping the blood sugar more even, as opposed to a seesaw effect whereby the blood sugar goes up after a big meal and then goes down when nothing is eaten for several hours in between. Try putting a 45-minute window around all the fruits you ingest to allow them to completely digest.

Question: What other types of aerobic exercises can I do if I want to vary my program and do more than just walking?

Answer: Other aerobic activities that you might want to try to vary your routine a little are bicycling or riding a stationary bike, skipping rope, Roller-blading, or jogging. If you are over 198 pounds, I don't recommend that you bicycle for more than 15 to 20 minutes at a time. While working with athletic teams that used indoor stationary bikes, I discovered that men who weighed more than 195 could easily develop lower back pain or groin pain when sitting on a bicycle for longer than that. If you want to make an exercise bicycle a part of your aerobic routine, I suggest that you make a mini-circuit, alternating it with 10 to 15 minutes of jumping rope and 10 to 15 minutes of walking on a treadmill. Jumping rope is an excellent aerobic exercise, and one that the boxers I have worked with utilize as part of their strength- and stamina-building routine. When you ride a bicycle, always make sure that you stretch out the muscles at the top and sides of your hips both before and after.

You can Rollerblade for 45 to 60 minutes a day, but be sure to wear a protective helmet, knee pads, elbow pads, and wrist guards.

Aerobic walking can easily progress to jogging. Make sure you are wearing the proper footgear since there is a difference in design and construction between walking shoes and running shoes due to the higher stress demands on the foot and joints during the latter form of exercise. If you are unused to running, I suggest starting out slowly, alternating longer and longer periods of jogging with your walking until you can run for 45 minutes to an hour. If you weigh more than 250 pounds, alternate running with other aerobic activities to prevent shin splints or stress fractures. As with all aerobic exercises, use the talk test to make sure that you are performing within your optimum fat-burning zone.

Question: Can I do the abdominal exercises daily if I want to? Or do I need some recovery time in between to allow my body to repair itself?

Answer: While it is true that you should usually allow at least a day between your overall body workouts with weights or exercise equipment at the gym to give your muscle tissue time to repair itself, you can do these abdominal exercises every day if you want to. As the support system for the core area of the body, these muscles—the spinal erectors, the abdominal muscles (erectus, transverse, and oblique), the gluteal muscles, the quadriceps, and the hamstrings—are all designed to work hard, so they can absorb the extra workouts. I do recommend, however, that you start slowly and build up with these core exercises. It is never good to overdo exercise in the beginning. Give your body a chance to adjust, and then be aware of how it is responding.

Question: If I can't keep my shoulders on the floor when I am doing some of the exercises, what should I do?

Answer: Eventually, if you keep doing the floor exercises, your body will stretch out more. In the meantime, think in terms of finding *your* body's "neutral position," one from which you can maintain the normal curvature of your spine, and do the exercises easily, comfortably, and without pain. Research has shown that when athletes work in this neutral pelvic position, they are less likely to become injured. In fact, proper positioning of the spine, which promotes spinal endurance, is a greater protector against injury than strength.

If your shoulder lifts up off the floor when your knees are touching it, place folded thicknesses of towel or a pillow under your shoulder. This will elevate the shoulder and give you a firm support while you are doing the movement. In any exercises where you are lying flat on your back, if you find that your neck or lower back is arched, you may also wish to put a folded towel under each of those areas for support. These aids will help you to have a "soft leverage" until your body stretches out.

Question: If I do this program, does that mean that I can't do any other types of exercises?

Answer: This program is specifically designed to work with any other exercise program that you are currently doing. When Stan began this program, he was already doing at least 45 minutes of exercises designed specifically for golfers. It was quite easy for him to combine the two programs for maximum benefit.

My exercises are designed primarily to tone and firm the love handle area, the core area of the body. If you want an overall body workout, I encourage you to combine my program with free weight training, circuit training in the gym, or any other overall exercise program that appeals to you.

For many years, losing weight in the love handle area has been a struggle for men. Even those who go to the gym regularly, including the six men I write about in chapter 6 who took part in this study, have found this area the toughest to reduce. It doesn't matter how "fit" you think you are. Top athletes I've worked with in professional boxing, the NFL, and professional baseball also have trouble keeping the love handle area toned and firm. But now, with the help of recent medical research, the glycemic index, and state-of-the-art core exercises, I've found a way to beat abdominal fat and the many disease risks that accompany it. There are not many sure things in life. But if you are willing to give this program a minimum of an hour a day— 15 to 20 minutes for the exercises and 45 minutes for the aerobic walking or advanced aerobic training—and follow the low-glycemic nutrition plan, I guarantee that you will begin to see the inches in your waistline melt away. Not only that, but you will feel better, have more energy, and live longer. So, what are you waiting for? Let's get out there and lose those love handles!

RESOURCES

Exercise Equipment

CDM Medical
816 Ladera Drive
Fort Worth, Texas 76108
800-400-7542 (Office)
817-448-8701 (FAX)
www.cdmsport.com
(sells Swiss balls, medicine balls, and the chop
and lift tubing)

DKSA
1280 Route 7A
Manchester Center, Vermont 05255
800-217-5282 (Office)
802-362-0825 (FAX)
www.stretchout.com
(stretch out strap)

www.fitnesswholesale.com
330-929-7227
(stretch straps and chop and lift tubing)

Nutrition

American Dietetic Association (ADA)
216 West Jackson Boulevard
Chicago, IL 60606
800-877-1600; 312-899-0040; 312-899-
4739 (FAX)
800-366-1655 (Consumer Hotline)
www.eatright.org
E-mails: infocenter@eatright.org

American Heart Association (AHA)
National Center
7272 Greenville Avenue
Dallas, TX 75231
800-242-8721

American Society for Clinical Nutrition (ASCN)
9650 Rockville Pike
Bethesda, MD 20814
301-530-7110;
301-571-1863 (FAX)
E-mail: secretar@acsn.faseb.org

149

The Glycemic Research Institute
601 Pennsylvania Avenue, N.W., Suite 900
Washington, D.C. 20004
202-434-8270
www.glycemic.com
www.anndeweesallen.com

Personal Edge Performance Nutrition
Nutritious Foods, Inc.
P.O. Box 88940
St. Louis, MO 63188
(877) 982-EDGE (3343)
(314) 982-3342 (FAX)
www.personaledgeprotein.com

Organizations

American College of Sports Medicine (ACSM)
P.O. Box 1440
Indianapolis, IN 46206-1440
(317) 637-9200
www.acsm.org

American Council on Exercise (ACE)
5820 Oberlin Drive, Suite 102
San Diego, CA 92121-3787
(619) 535-8227
www.acefitness.org

Cooper Institute for Aerobic Research (CIAR)
12330 Preston Road
Dallas, TX 75230
(214) 701-8001
www.cooperinst.org

Shape Up America!
6707 Democracy Boulevard, Suite 306
Bethesda, MD 20817
(301) 493-5368
www.shapeup.org

Books

Fight Fat After Forty by Pamela Peeke, M.D., M.P.H.
(Viking Press, 2000)

The Glucose Revolution: The Authoritative Guide to the Glycemic Index by Jennie Brand-Miller, Ph.D., Thomas M.S. Wolever, M.D., Ph.D., Stephen Colagiuri, M.D., and Kaye Foster-Powell, (Marlowe and Co. 1999)

The New Millennium Diet Revolution by Keith De Orio, M.D., with Robert Dursi, C.N.M. (Prominence Publishers 2000)

Additional Online Resources

Ask Dr. Weil [Andrew Weil, M.D.]
www.drweil.com

Center for Anxiety and Stress Treatment
www.stressrelease.com

Health Net
www.healthnet.com

The Institute for Stress Management
www.hyperstress.com

My Personal Web Page
www.mackieshilstone.com

Omega Institute for Holistic Studies
www.omega-inst.org

Ochsner Clinic and Hospital
www.ochsner.org

Yoga Journal
www.yogajournal.com

*on*health
www.onhealth.com

INDEX

Page numbers
in *italic* indicate
illustrations; those in
bold indicate tables.

ABOUT THE AUTHOR

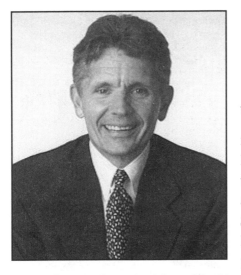

When Michael Spinks made history by becoming the *only* light-heavyweight boxer to successfully win the world heavyweight boxing title against Larry Holmes, he had Mackie Shilstone to thank. When baseball legend Darryl Strawberry needed to salvage a plummeting career with the San Francisco Giants, he turned to Mackie for help. When international superstar Chuck Norris decided to redesign his training routine and strengthen his body for a starring role in a film, he went to Mackie. When all-star Ozzie Smith, at the age of 30, wanted just 3 more years on the baseball diamond with the St. Louis Cardinals, he put his performance training in the hands of Mackie. His career continued another 11 years until he retired at the age of 41. Three months after baseball star Brett Butler had surgery and radiation treatment for lymphatic

ʒer, he put in 17 days of rigorous training with Mackie and made a miracu-
lous comeback with the Dodgers.

Mackie Shilstone is one of America's most influential sports performance
managers, whose expertise has played a pivotal role in the success and
longevity of scores of million-dollar world-class athletes. Over 1,000 professional athletes to date have turned to Mackie to give them the body, the
drive, the stamina, and the performance they need to win. Mackie has also
transformed the lives of hundreds of everyday people struggling with
weight problems, poor nutrition, and lack of motivation. To Mackie, there
are no barriers between professional athletes and the average person, only
different target goals and differing training times to reach those goals.

With a master's degree in both nutrition and business administration,
Mackie is the Executive Director of the Center for Performance
Enhancement and Lifestyle Management at the Elmwood Fitness Center, a
division of Ochsner Clinic and Hospital. This is the only program of its kind
in the world, centered on Mackie's unique, cutting-edge expertise. He is a
clinical instructor of public health and preventative medicine at Louisiana
State University and is currently a special advisor to the United States
Olympic Committee on sports nutrition and a member of the Governor's
Council on Physical Fitness and Sports.

The author of *Feelin' Good About Fitness* (Pelican Publishing, 1986), and
*Lose Your Love Handles: A 3-Step Program to Streamline Your Waist in Only 30
Days* (Perigee, 2001), Mackie has also written articles for prestigious health
and fitness journals such as the *American Medical Athletic Association
Quarterly* and *The Physiologist*.

The astonishing results of Mackie's work with top athletes are constantly reported in magazines and newspapers across the country.

Over 1,000 articles, appearing in print media such as the *Wall Street
Journal*, the *New York Times*, the *Los Angeles Times*, *USA Today*, *People* magazine, and *Inc.*, have praised the Mackie Shilstone method. *KO Magazine*
voted him among the top 50 Most Influential People in the history of boxing.

Mackie has also appeared on most of the major news shows in the country including *ESPN*, *The Today Show*, *HBO*, and *Good Morning America*. On a
48 Hours' exposé of the diet industry, Mackie was heralded as "the weight
control guru for top athletes in the country."

Mackie also appears weekly on *The Morning Show*, the highest rated show
of its kind in the country, which has an audience of 30,000 viewers. This program is broadcast on WWL, the highest rated per capita CBS affiliate in the

nation. Examples of his segments, which are always changing, in
"Fitness Kitchen," which offers healthy recipes to viewers, and "Yoga with
Mackie and Meg." Mackie's segments are also shown on *The Morning Show*
Web site on the Internet, WWLTV.com, which receives 30,000 hits per month.

Monday through Friday 4,500 listeners in New Orleans, and thousands of
others throughout Louisiana and Mississippi, hear Mackie on his call-in
radio program *The Mackie Shilstone Show,* broadcast on WSMB (1350
AM). *Mackie's Health Minute* is heard by 122,000 listeners nationwide,
twice a day during drivetime at 6:15 A.M. and 6:15 P.M. on WSMB's sis-
ter station WWL (870 AM) the 2nd largest 50,000 watt station in the
country.

Mackie is currently the sports medicine coordinator for the New Orleans
Brass, an East Coast Hockey League team. He is chairman of the Mayor's
Advisory Board on Physical Fitness for the City of New Orleans.